WORLD BANK WORKING PAPER NO. 192

Incentives and Dynamics in the Ethiopian Health Worker Labor Market

William Jack
Joose de Laat
Kara Hanson
Agnes Soucat

Africa Region Human Development Department

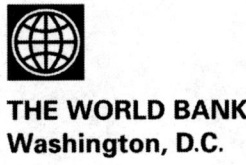

THE WORLD BANK
Washington, D.C.

ISBN: 978-0-8213-8358-2
eISBN: 978-0-8213-8364-3
ISSN: 1726-5878   DOI: 10.1596/978-0-8213-8358-2

Library of Congress Cataloging-in-Publication Data has been requested.

Contents

Foreword

By international standards, the supply of health workers in Ethiopia is low. In addition, those who do enter the profession and remain in the country disproportionately live and work in the capital city, Addis Ababa. This story is repeated across the developing world, and in particular in Sub-Saharan Africa, where shortages of health workers are deemed chronic. Increasing the supply of health workers, and improving their geographic distribution, requires an understanding of their responsiveness to changes in the incentives and constraints they face, and the efficacy with which labor markets can be expected to allocate scarce human resources for health (HRH).

This book presents evidence on these and other HRH issues from a new survey of Ethiopian health workers. Detailed data was collected from nearly 1,000 health workers which is used to answer some fundamental questions: (i) how do compensation levels vary with location, training, experience, etc.?; (ii) what kinds of incentive packages are potentially most effective in attracting workers to under-served rural areas?; and (iii) what can we learn about the health worker labor market from one of its unique institutional features, that is, that new graduates are assigned to their first jobs via a lottery?

The rigorous study methodology and policy relevant findings may be of interest to all those working to improve the allocation of human resources for health in the developing world. Ethiopia for one, has shown strong government commitment to the development of its health workforce, and is determined to futher refine and strengthen policies to serve the poor. Evidence on what motivates doctors and nurses to practice in remote rural areas will support the government design and refine targeted interventions on HRH that will accellerate progress towards the MDGs even further.

Yaw Ansu,
Sector Director, Human Development
Africa Region
World Bank

Acknowledgements

This work was produced by the HRH Team of the Africa Region Health Systems for Outcomes (HSO) Program of the World Bank and was made possible by the contributions of a large number of individuals and organizations. Financial support from the Bill and Melinda Gates Foundation and NORAD is gratefully recognized. We thank Dr Tedros, Dr Kebede, and Dr Nejmudinthe of the Ministry of Health, and the Government of Ethiopia. Other contributors include Dr. Aklilu Kidanu and colleagues from the Miz-Hasab Research Center in Addis Ababa, as well as Christopher H. Herbst, Magnus Lindlow, Gebreselassie Okubagzhi, Pieter Serneels, and Kate Tulenko from the World Bank.

Abstract

By international standards, the supply of health workers in Ethiopia is tiny. In addition, those who do enter the profession and remain in the country disproportionately live and work in the capital, Addis Ababa. This book examines the incentives and constraints faced by health workers when choosing where to work, the likely responses of workers to alternative incentive packages, and the longer-term performance of the health worker labor market.

Acronyms and Abbreviations

DCE	Discrete Choice Experiments
HIV/AIDS	Human immunodeficiency virus/acquired immunodeficiency syndrome
HRH	Human Resources for Health
HSO	Health Systems for Outcomes
MoH	Ministry of Health
MRS	Marginal rate of substitution
NGO	Nongovernmental organization
NNM	Nearest neighbor matching
NRMP	National Resident Matching Program
OLS	Ordinary Least Squares
SNNPR	Southern Nations, Nationalities, and Peoples Region
SPSS	Scalable Stream Processing Systems
WHO	World Health Organization

CHAPTER 1

Studying the Health Labor Market in Ethiopia: An Overview

Joost de Laat, Kara Hanson, William Jack, Aklilu Kidanu, and Agnes Soucat

Introduction

The supply and geographic distribution of health workers are major constraints to improving health in low-income countries. A number of recent studies have highlighted the shortage of skilled health workers in many settings (World Health Organization [WHO], 2006), the impact this has on health outcomes (Anand and Barnighausen, 2004), and the risk this poses for the achievement of the Millenium Development Goals (WHO, 2006; Joint Learning Initiative, 2004). However, there remains limited evidence about what sorts of policies will attract nurses and doctors into medical training, improve the retention of trained health workers, and encourage them to work in rural areas where problems of inaccessibility of services are most acute.

The challenges of human development are particularly extreme in Ethiopia, a country with a population of over 70 million people, 85% of whom live in rural areas. It is one of the poorest countries in the world, with per capita income of about $150, and although the poverty rate has fallen by 8 percentage points over the last 10 years, it nonetheless remained at 37% in 2006. The country faces acute challenges in reaching all of the Millenium Development Goals, including the three goals relating to health—to reduce child mortality, improve maternal health, and combat HIV/AIDS, malaria, and other diseases. In 2005 the infant mortality rate was 77 per 1,000, the under-5 mortality rate was 123 per 1,000, and the maternal mortality rate was 673 per 100,000. In 2006 about half of all mothers received some kind of antenatal service, and 15% of deliveries were attended by a health worker. Ethiopia has escaped the ravages of HIV/AIDS compared with other countries in Africa, and had an adult prevalence of 2.1% in 2006.

With an eye to informing the policy making process, this report summarizes the methodology and findings of a study of the health labor market conducted in Ethiopia in 2007. We first discuss the prevailing human resources setting in the health sector. This is followed by a description of the empirical methodology, including survey design and sampling issues, and presentation of summary statistics on the workforce and its demographic and economic characteristics. We then present two separate analyses using the data collected. First, we estimate the relationships between job assignments and career development, with special attention to the institutional mechanisms that characterize the health sector labor market—in particular distinguishing between the lottery system used to assign jobs to new graduates, and what we refer to as the market. Second, we estimate the expected labor supply responses to a variety of financial and in-kind incentives that might be provided in order to attract workers to rural areas.

We group our findings into three categories: descriptive, analytic, and predictive. Among the descriptive results, the most striking is the extent to which health worker salaries and incomes vary geographically. In Addis Ababa, doctors earn 50% more than they would on average in Tigray and the Southern Nations, Nationalities, and Peoples Region (SNNPR) if they work in the public sector, and on average three times as much if they work in the private sector. Of course, some of this reflects different characteristics—such as age, experience, specialization, and other factors. Half of private sector doctors in Addis own a car, while fewer than 2% of SNNPR physicians do so.

Our analytic results focus mainly on the physician labor market. They include an analysis of the effects of job choices and assignments early in a physician's career, including the long-term career consequences of taking a job in the regions, and the long-term effects of participating in the lottery system itself. We present evidence that the labor market for physicians who took part in the lottery operates *less efficiently* than for physicians who did not participate in the lottery. We rationalize this by suggesting that the lottery obfuscates information about physician quality, which would be valuable to future employers, and this imperfection of information leads to adverse selection in the labor market.

Finally, our predictive results are based on a discrete choice experiment that was part of our questionnaire. This component of the study enables us to estimate the value that doctors and nurses place on different job attributes, and how they vary across individuals. We find, for example, that doubling wages in areas outside the capital would increase the share of doctors willing to work there from about 7% to more than 50%. Providing high-quality housing would increase physician labor supply to about 27%, which is equivalent to paying a wage bonus of about 46%. Doubling wages paid to nurses for work in rural areas outside cities increases their labor supply from 4% to 27%, while the non-wage attribute that is most effective in inducing them to relocate to rural areas is the quality of equipment and drugs. The same impact could be achieved by increasing rural nursing wages by about 57% for men and 69% for women.

Human Resources for Health in Ethiopia

This section provides background information on human resources in the health sector, and a description of the institutional structure of the health labor market.

Human Resources

This section reviews the size and distribution of the health workforce in Ethiopia. The Ministry of Health (MoH 2005) reports that in 2005 there were a total of 2,453 physicians in the country, of which 444 (17%) operated in the private sector, 578 (23%) in the nongovernmental organization (NGO) sector, and 354 (14%) in other government organizations (such as the military). As reported in Table 1.1, 42% of physicians are specialists (1,067 out of 2,543).

Of the 830 physicians classified as "public," 20% were located in Addis Ababa. Although the Ministry of Health reports the distribution of public doctors, data on the geographic distribution of *all* doctors is not readily available. Table 1.2 reports the geographic pattern of physicians and ratios of population to physicians. The ratios of population to *all* physicians reported in the third column are calculated under the strong assumption that the geographic distribution of non-public physicians is the same as that of public physicians. Even under this very conservative assumption, the average population-to-physician ratio is fully seven times higher across the five most populous regions (where 92% of the population live) than it is in Addis Ababa.

If the distribution of non-public physicians is skewed towards Addis Ababa, then the disparity between the capital and the regions increases. Of particular importance in this

Table 1.1. Physicians by Sector and Type

	Specialists	GPs	Total
Public	240	590	830
Central	164	83	247
NGOs	270	308	578
OGOs	178	176	354
Private	215	229	444
Total	1,067	1,386	2,453

Source: Ministry of Health, 2005.

regard is the private sector, which has grown rapidly in recent years, with the vast majority of this growth occurring in Addis Ababa. Figure 1.1 uses the MoH 2005 data to compare the geographic distribution of public doctors, with that of public and private doctors, assuming that all private doctors work in Addis. In this case, nearly half of the doctors (48%) worked in Addis in 2005, home to 4% of the population.

According to survey data we collected in 2007 on physicians in Ethiopia, 380 out of an estimated 597 physicians working in Addis (or 63%) currently work as physicians outside the public sector, the vast majority in the private sector. In one of the two other regions covered by the survey, in the SNNPR, about 10% of physicians are estimated to be working outside the public sector (including NGOs). In the second surveyed region, Tigray, virtually all doctors are believed to work in the public sector.

Against this background, the World Health Organization recommends a population-physician ratio of 10,000 to 1. The last row of Table 1.2 reports the country *average* population-physician ratio to be about three times this level, suggesting that the first challenge facing Ethiopia is to train and retain enough doctors to triple the workforce. However, an equally

Table 1.2. Geographic Distribution of Physicians, 2005

Region	Number *public* physicians	Ratio of population to *public* physicians	Ratio of population to *all* physicians*
Addis Ababa (4.0%)	**167**	**17,291**	**5,851**
Larger regions (92.2%)	**555**	**121,395**	**41,075**
Oromia (35.3%)	186	138,802	46,965
Amhara (25.5%)	131	142,184	48,109
SNNPR (19.8%)	106	136,695	46,252
Tigray (5.8%)	77	88,004	18,557
Somali (5.8%)	55	76,696	25,951
Smaller regions (3.8%)	**108**	**25,756**	**8,716**
Afar (1.9%)	17	79,925	27,043
Ben Gumuz (0.8%)	14	43,536	14,731
Dire Dawa (0.5%)	30	12,784	4,326
Gambella (0.3%)	6	40,066	13,557
Hareri (0.3%)	41	4,623	1,564
Total	830	88,004	29,777

* This column assumes that all non-public doctors are distributed in the same proportion as public physicians.

Source: Ministry of Health, 2005.

Figure 1.1. Geographic distribution of "public" doctors and "public plus private" doctors.

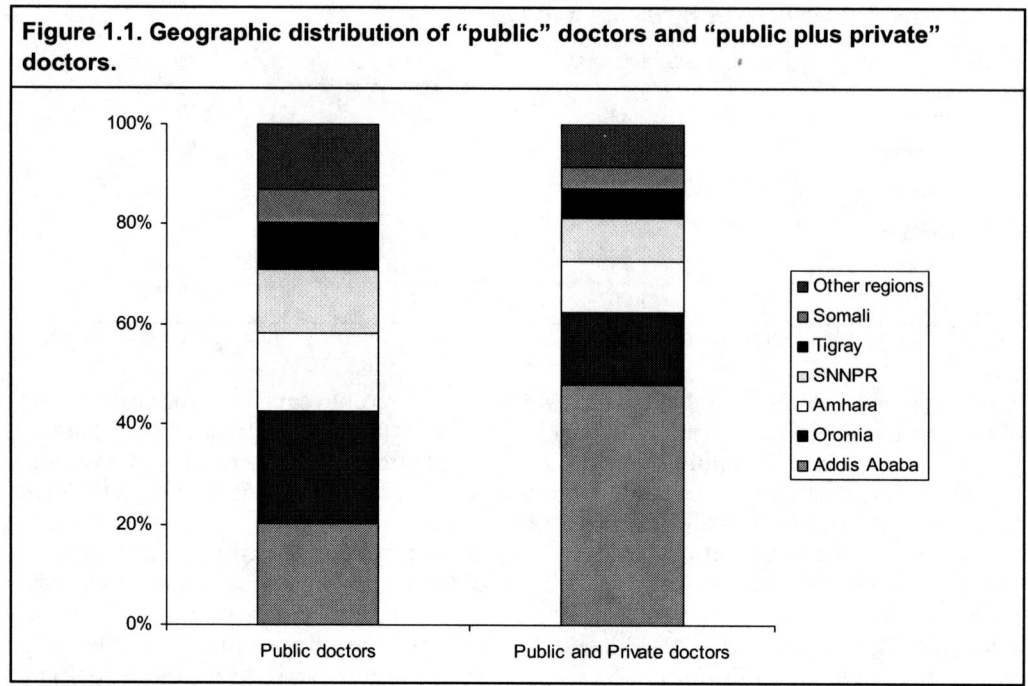

Source: Ministry of Health, 2005.

pressing concern, and one that must be addressed if the WHO-recommended ratios are to be met in a meaningful way, is the paucity of physicians in rural areas. Training more doctors who end up working in the capital or overseas will have little impact on the availability of health care services for most people, and arguably little impact on health outcomes. With ratios of 40 to 50 thousand people per doctor in the largest regions, there is an overwhelming need to attract medical providers to rural areas, and to get them to stay.

The Lottery System

The primary vehicle through which the Ethiopian health system has ensured a supply of health workers to the rural regions is a kind of national clearing house. Each year a national lottery is announced through the media in September. Health workers who graduated in the previous June and July, as well as doctors who have completed their internships, are invited to go to the Ministry of Health, starting in October, to participate in the lottery.

Under the lottery system—which is officially mandatory, although in practice appears to be optional—a participant is randomly assigned to one of the twelve regions of the country, and the regional health bureau is informed of this assignment. Job assignments at the regional level are administrated by the relevant regional bureau (World Bank, 2006). Assigned workers are required to serve a fixed number of years before being "released" and permitted to apply for other positions.[1]

We estimate that about 60% of physicians currently working in Ethiopia participated in the lottery. While the lottery is still officially in place, during the past five years Ethiopia has embarked on a radical decentralization program across all areas of the public sector, with much of the responsibility for service delivery being devolved to lower levels of government, and allowing private health facilities to operate alongside public ones. According to discussions with senior health officials, legal questions have also been raised about the government's ability to enforce the requirement that doctors whose training was federally funded can be required to work for a fixed period in a job assigned through the lottery.

In what follows, we use the lottery system to estimate the long-term impacts of rural assignment, and compare the effect of getting a job in Addis early in a doctor's career on later labor market outcomes among lottery participants and non-participants. We then examine whether participation in the lottery itself can compromise the efficiency of future allocations in the physician labor market.

Empirical Methodology

In early 2007 a survey of physicians and nurses was undertaken by an Addis Ababa-based research firm, the Miz-Hasab Research Institute. Health workers at hospitals and health centers in Addis, Tigray, and the SNNPR were interviewed and asked about their work, careers, incomes, families, training, experiences, and other employment-related issues. They were also asked to provide information on the value they placed on different attributes of their jobs, including location, facility quality, etc. The results of this survey are presented later in this chapter. In this section we review the sampling strategy and the nature of the questionnaires.

Sampling

Our sampling strategy aimed at obtaining representative samples of doctors and nurses from three of Ethiopia's eleven regions—the capital city of Addis Ababa, Tigray, and the SNNPR, as illustrated in Figure 1.2.

Addis is a city of about 3 million people and is located in the central highlands. Tigray has a population of about 4 million people and lies in the extreme north of the country, bordering Eritrea. The SNNPR, with a population of 14 million, borders Kenya to

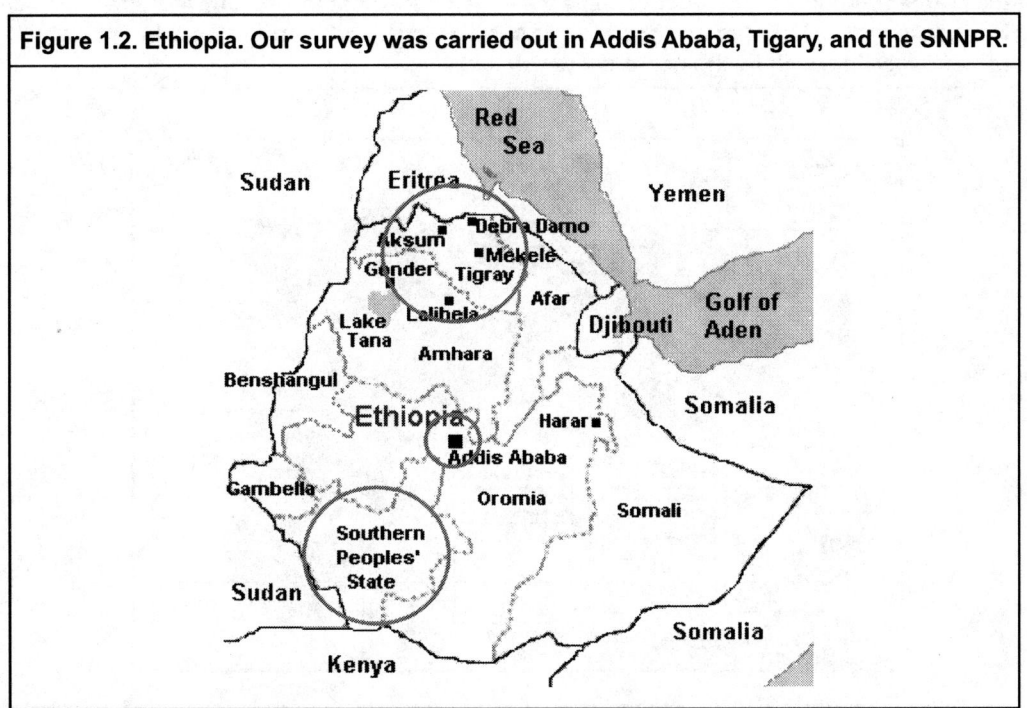

Figure 1.2. Ethiopia. Our survey was carried out in Addis Ababa, Tigary, and the SNNPR.

the south. Our sample is representative within these geographic areas.[2] The design over-sampled doctors in the SNNPR and Tigray, due to the small number of doctors outside Addis Ababa; all doctors in these rural regions were sampled, while only about one third of doctors in Addis were. Our final sample included 219 doctors and 645 nurses working in health centers and hospitals. Detailed sampling information is illustrated for Tigray and the SNNPR in Figures 1.3 and 1.4.

A random sample of one third of doctors was achieved in Addis Ababa by (a) randomly sampling facilities of the various types with sampling weights corresponding to the estimated proportion of doctors working across the different facilities; and (b) interviewing all doctors at the sampled facilities. In the SNNPR and Tigray, all doctors were included in the sample. This was achieved by sampling all public hospitals in the SNNPR and Tigray. (There are generally no doctors in non-hospital health facilities in these regions, and there were no private hospitals.) In addition to interviewing health workers, we administered a facility-level survey with the facility administrator or other senior official at each facility we visited. A summary of our sample is provided in Table 1.3.

Among doctors, the interview response rate varied widely across regions. In Tigray it was very high (88%), while in the SNNPR and Addis Ababa it was lower—58% and 66%, respectively. In Addis, the response rates differed in public and private facilities. At public facilities, all doctors present agreed to be interviewed, although 40% of sampled doctors were absent on the day of the interview (28% for unexplained reasons and 12% for planned leave). However, at private facilities, no unexplained absences were recorded, while 18% of doctors were absent on planned leave. In contrast to public facilities, the share of sampled doctors who were present but refused to be interviewed was 27%. In Tigray, non-response arose because one sampled facility no longer existed, and one was inaccessible for security reasons, but at visited facilities absenteeism and refusal rates were very low. In the SNNPR,

Figure 1.3. Tigray sampling information. Each symbol H represents a hospital in the corresponding woreda. All hospitals were visited (except for the one in Kafta Humera woreda). The blue and green stars show woredas with and without hospitals, respectively, in which health centers were visited.

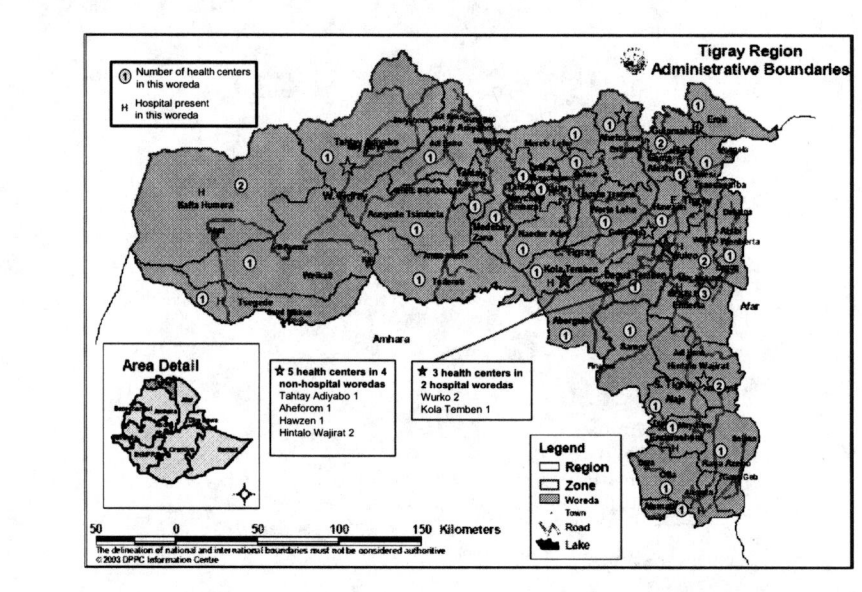

Figure 1.4. SNNPR sampling information. Each symbol H represents a hospital in the corresponding woreda. All hospitals were visited. The blue and green stars show woredas with and without hospitals, respectively, in which health centers were visited. Non-hospital woredas were clustered.

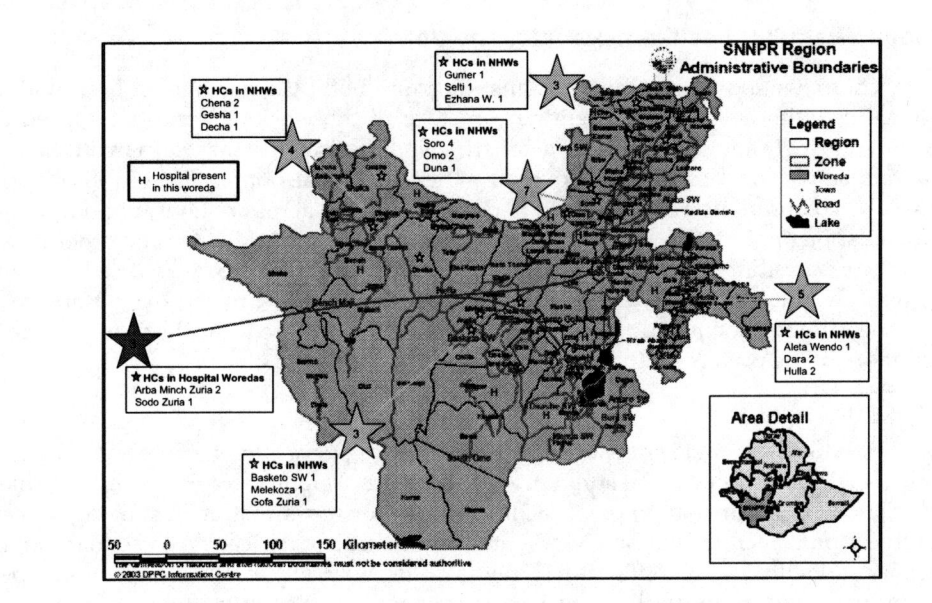

42% of doctors listed as being employed were absent at the time of the facility visit, although 9 out of 10 of them were reported as being absent for training purposes.

Survey Instrument

Our survey instrument included three components.[3] The first was a short questionnaire administered to the director or other senior administrative officer of the facility visited; this concerned facility-level information. The other two components were administered to each health worker interviewed. Of these, the first component asked for information about (i) lottery participation and characteristics of the worker's first job, (ii) work history, (iii) training, (iv) current income-earning activities, and (v) household characteristics and

Table 1.3. Numbers of Facilities and Health Workers Surveyed, by Region

	Addis Ababa	SNNPR	Tigray	Total
Facilities	40	39	18	97
Hospitals	6	12	11	29
Health centers and clinics	34	27	7	68
Health workers	362	206	293	861
Doctors	91	72	56	219
Nurses	271	221	150	642

incomes. The second component of the individual questionnaire presented respondents with a number of hypothetical employment choices, from which we estimated the value of alternative job characteristics and how these valuations vary across different types of workers.

Descriptive Results: Facilities, People, and Jobs

In this section, we report summary statistics from both the facility and individual questionnaires, with a view to presenting a picture of the working conditions faced by health workers, their demographic characteristics, and the incomes they earn in alternative occupations, across the three regions coverd by the survey. The bottom line of this analysis is that working conditions do not appear to differ markedly across regions, although they are somewhat better, in some respects, in the private sector in Addis. On the other hand, health workers are different across regions—they are more likely to be married in some places, to be women in others, and of different ages in others. But the big difference is money, especially for doctors: doctors are paid significantly more in Addis than outside— and still more in the private sector in Addis.

Facility Conditions

Table 1.4 provides summary statistics from the facility survey for facilities at which at least one physician worked.[4] The summary statistics are weighted by the estimated share of physicians working in each type of facility. The table shows that at least along several measurable inputs, facilities in the SNNPR and Tigray are not noticably worse than public facilities in Addis. In fact, SNNPR and Tigray facilities with physicians are better equiped to test for HIV and are more likely to have sufficient water supply. However, there are differences between the two regions outside Addis. For example, only half the doctors in Tigray work in facilities with sufficient medicine, compared with 73% and 88% of those in Addis and the SNNPR, respectively. Similarly, Tigray has more inpatient beds per doctor and more outpatients than both the SNNPR and public facilities in Addis.

On the other hand, private facilities in Addis are much smaller, with about half the number of inpatients and outpatients per doctor, compared with public facilities in the capital. Some quality indicators, such as water availability, are reported as significantly better in Addis' private facilities, but in other areas, private facilities report being either no better (equipment) or somewhat worse (medicine).

The SNNPR and Tigray are both remote areas of Ethiopia. Although Tigray is further from Addis, doctors working in the SNNPR are more remote in terms of their travel times to the regional capital—it takes an average of 6 hours to reach the regional capital, Awassa, compared with 5.1 hours for doctors in Tigray to reach that region's capital, Mekele. This reflects the fact that the SNNPR covers a much larger geographic area.

Table 1.5 presents information relating to facility conditions and work environments as reported by individual health workers (and not by the administrator of the facility). We highlight two particular differences in work envoirnment between public and private facilities. First, both doctors and nurses are much less likely to report being overworked in private facilities: 22% and 20% of private doctors and nurses, respectively, report that there is often not enough time to complete tasks, compared with sample averages of 55% and 48%; and fully 6% of private doctors report that idle time is common in their jobs, compared with a sample average of 2%. Secondly, the degree of supervision seems higher in private facilities, in both "carrot" and "stick" forms. That is, the shares of doctors and nurses reporting supportive supervision, 62% and 69% (respectively), are significantly higher than the sample averages (45% and 46%); and the shares that say their supervisor reprimands staff (36% and 49%) are also higher than the sample averages (31% and 40%).

Table 1.4. Facility-Level Information, Based on Interviews with an Administrator, for Facilities with at Least One Physician

	All surveyed regions	Addis Ababa		SNNPR	Tigray
		Public	Private*		
Number of sampled facilities (with at least one physician)	77	8	31	21**	17
Facility size					
Number of doctors	834	217	380	189	48
Doctors per facility	3.8 (4.9)	6.9 (10.6)	2.6 (2.4)	5.2 (4.8)	2.6 (2.2)
Number inpatient beds	79.5 (91.7)	141.5 (112.2)	21.5 (40.1)	114.5 (63.5)	121.3 (105.6)
Number inpatient beds per doctor	20.9	20.5	8.3	22.0	46.7
Number outpatients	104.4 (93.3)	181.5 (86.9)	38.0 (43.0)	139.8 (77.0)	143.9 (106.8)
Number outpatients per doctor	27.5	26.3	14.6	26.9	55.3
Hours travel to regional capital	—	—	—	6.0 (5.5)	5.3 (5.0)
Facility conditions (%)					
Reliable electricity/phone	99.3	100.0	100.0	97.4	97.9
Functioning X-ray machine	91.3	77.0	81.6	85.2	83.3
Functioning laboratory	100.0	100.0	100.0	100.0	100.0
Functioning operating theatre	62.1	61.8	42.6	92.6	97.9
Equipment to test for HIV	83.6	66.4	86.8	92.6	100.0
Sufficient water supply	74.5	23.0	96.0	87.3	85.4
Sufficient medicine	79.1	88.5	72.9	88.4	50.0
Sufficient equipment	87.1	83.9	84.5	100.0	70.8

* Includes for-profit and non-profit NGO and missionary facilities.

** Includes 3 private facilities.

Statistics are calculated using frequency weights corresponding to total number of doctors by region working in (1) public hospitals, (2) private hospitals, (3) government health centers, and (4) private, NGO, or missionary clinics.

The data also allow us to identify differences between the assessments made by physicians and nurses regarding their work environments. There do not appear to be systematic differences between reports of the two types of health workers, except in two cases. First, in terms of workload, the share of physicians who report that there is often not sufficient time to complete their tasks consistently exceeds the share of nurses who report the same thing, especially in the public sector. Staff appear most overworked on average in the SNNPR, but the difference between doctors' and nurses' perceptions is largest in Tigray.

Demographic Information

Demographic data from the individual-level questionnaires are reported in Table 1.6. Doctors in Addis Ababa, especially those working in the private sector, are older and more

Table 1.5. Facility-Level Information, Based on Interviews with Individual Health Workers

Facility conditions	All regions		Addis Ababa				SNNPR		Tigray	
			Public		Private*					
	Doc	Nurse	Doc	Nurse	Doc	Nurse	Doc	Nurse	Doc	Nurse
Availability of supplies (%)										
Soap	75.0	69.0	68.7	69.1	100	100	63.8	59.7	53.5	67.1
Water	75.0	75.2	82.5	79.9	98.0	100	59.0	61.8	44.2	77.2
Plastic gloves	88.7	85.7	84.3	84.8	100	100	92.2	84.3	68.6	82.8
Facial mask	58.7	43.0	57.8	51.8	88.9	92.5	49.1	32.1	16.2	23.5
Sterile syringes	93.7	91.8	91.1	92.1	100	100	94.7	92.1	84.4	87.2
Medicines	73.9	70.9	61.3	76.1	97.8	91.3	79.3	73.0	42.2	50.8
Physical condition of facility (%)										
Good	43.4	40.9	30.3	24.2	58.0	79.8	39.3	37.0	40.7	46.3
Fair	42.1	45.6	48.5	53.2	38.0	18.6	38.5	51.6	45.4	41.6
Bad	14.5	13.5	21.2	22.6	4.0	1.6	22.2	11.4	14.0	12.1
Work environment										
Workload (%)										
Often not time to do tasks	55.1	48.2	67.3	58.2	22.0	20.3	82.1	61.2	61.6	31.5
Usually time to do tasks	43.0	51.1	32.7	40.4	72.0	79.8	18.0	38.8	38.4	67.1
Idle time common	2.0	0.6	0.0	1.0	6.0	0.0	0.0	0.0	0.0	1.3
Supervision (%)										
Supervisor reprimands	31.1	40.3	34.7	39.5	36.0	49.0	34.2	38.8	12.8	38.9
Supervisor supportive	45.3	46.1	32.0	38.3	62.0	68.8	50.4	45.2	26.7	45.0

* Includes for-profit and non-profit NGO and missionary facilities

experienced than those in the regions. Men are over-represented in the private sector in Addis, while the SNNPR has virtually no female doctors. The doctors in our sample come from large families—on average they have 6.4 siblings. But they have relatively small families of their own—on average they have 1 child. Nurses have more children, on average. Only one third of doctors and one half of nurses in SNNPR are married, but although marriage is most common among doctors in Addis (61% and 74% in the public and private sectors, respectively, compared with 45% in Tigray), nurses are more likely to be married in Tigray (79%, compared with 65% in Addis). Similarly, about 50% of doctors have no children, but this share ranges from 28% among private-sector physicians in Addis to over 80% in the SNNPR. Among those doctors and nurses with children, the average numbers are 2.1 and 2.7, and there is relatively little difference across regions.

Table 1.6. Demographic Characteristics of Sampled Health Workers

| Demographics | Doctors | | | | | Nurses | | | | |
| | All | Addis | | SNNPR | Tigray | All | Addis | | SNNPR | Tigray |
		Public	Private				Public	Private		
Share female (%)	17.1	30.0	16.0	2.6	26.8	64.3	73.8	84.4	52.1	61.8
Share married (%)	55.5	61.3	74.0	33.3	45.2	63.3	65.3	65.5	50.2	79.3
Age (years)	36.1	39.2	41.2	29.3	31.5	33.4	34.5	35.3	31.0	34.7
	(0.90)	(1.64)	(1.78)	(1.16)	(1.61)	(0.49)	(0.73)	(0.86)	(1.25)	(0.71)
Number of siblings	6.4	6.1	6.5	6.4	6.6	6.5	6.4	6.7	6.5	6.3
	(0.19)	(0.31)	(0.37)	(0.26)	(0.62)	(0.12)	(0.21)	(0.39)	(0.22)	(0.18)
Number of children	1.01	0.90	1.68	0.44	0.71	1.56	1.26	1.32	1.48	2.14
	(0.11)	(0.14)	(0.22)	(0.22)	(0.20)	(0.12)	(0.09)	(0.16)	(0.27)	(0.17)
Share with no children (%)	52.6	48.5	28.0	82.1	61.6	42.5	44.3	44.9	53.8	22.7
Number of children (for those with)	2.14	1.75	2.33	2.48	1.85	2.72	2.26	2.40	3.22	2.77
	(0.15)	(0.15)	(0.23)	(0.54)	(0.20)	(0.11)	(0.09)	(0.22)	(0.25)	(0.13)
Family connections to profession (%)										
Parents health workers	1.8	5.2	0.0	0.85	2.3	5.1	6.8	5.9	5.2	2.7
Siblings health workers	18.2	14.8	18.0	20.5	19.8	19.5	22.2	28.5	17.2	15.3
Other family health workers	18.5	19.9	26.0	13.7	7.0	15.7	18.2	22.5	14.9	10.7
Live in same region as at age 10	50.2	44.1	42.0	53.0	75.6	63.8	35.6	34.2	74.7	93.3
Type of job (%)										
Primary job in the private sector	36.9	0	100	9.4	0.0	14.0	0	100	5.4	0.0
Specialist	27.8	40.4	38.0	6.8	19.8	—	—	—	—	—

We find evidence that doctors are more likely to have moved away from their home region to Addis than to either of the regions. This is reflected in the fact that 75% of those in Tigray reported having lived there at age 10, compared with 50% in the SNNPR, and about 41% in Addis. These data suggest two competing interpretations: either it is more difficult to get health workers to move to Tigray than to the SNNPR, or natives of Tigray are more inclined to stay in their home region than those of the SNNPR. The data on family structure tends to support the latter explanation.

While a sizeable share of health workers (about 18% of doctors and 19% of nurses) have siblings in the profession, there seems to be a surprisingly small intergenerational medical link. The link is most pronounced among public-sector doctors in Addis Ababa: 5.2 % of them report have parents who were health workers, compared to 1% and 2% in the SNNPR and Tigray. This could indicate that having a parent in the business makes it easier to find a public-sector job in Addis. If so, having such contacts seems to have no positive impact on a doctor's chance of getting a job in the private sector in Addis—none of the doctors in our sample with private-sector jobs in Addis had parents in the profession.

Finally, if regions outside Addis Ababa have difficulty attracting health workers in general, they find it even more problematic recruiting specialists.

Incomes

In economic terms, doctors in Addis do better than those in the. As reported in columns 3 and 4 of Table 1.7, asset ownership is higher in Addis, with one half and one quarter of the doctors working in private and public facilities (respectively) reporting ownership of a car, compared with less than 2% and 5% in the SNNPR and Tigray, respectively. House ownership is higher among private-sector physicians in Addis (35%), but the rates among other doctors are similar (10–16%). These patterns of asset ownership naturally match the patterns of earned incomes.

Doctors working in the public sector in Addis earn salaries about 50% more than the average doctor in the regions, while salaries of private-sector doctors are three times as much as those in Tigray and the SNNPR. Part of this differential likely reflects the advantages of experience (Addis doctors are older) and specialization (they are more likely to be specialized). However, we find that the rates of specialization in the public and private sectors in Addis are virtually identical, suggesting that training is not the sole driver of observed income differentials. Nurses in Addis earn significantly smaller premiums over regional salaries—about 14% more if they work in the public sector and 36% more in the private sector.

The gap between private-sector salaries in Addis and those of other doctors is partly offset by additional sources of income: public-sector doctors in Addis earn additional income equal to 21% of their salaries, while the figures in the SNNPR and Tigray are 17%

Table 1.7. Incomes and Assets of Sampled Health Workers

Income	Doctors					Nurses				
	All	Addis		SNNPR	Tigray	All	Addis		SNNPR	Tigray
		Public	Private				Public	Private		
Salary (US$)	284.5	244.6	480.5	156.4	176.6	100.9	106.8	128.3	87.7	100.8
	(17.4)	(10.5)	(39.0)	(14.8)	(13.9)	(2.0)	(2.1)	(9.6)	(2.7)	(1.96)
Other compensation with job (%)	52.7	29.3	46.0	85.5	53.5	47.0	15.5	35.9	73.3	48.7
Housing allowance (%)	18.9	0	0	52.1	34.8	5.9	0	0	11.7	6.7
Total income of health worker (US$)	320.9	297.0	496.8	181.4	233.1	102.6	109.3	130.1	87.7	103.7
	(24.8)	(24.8)	(40.1)	(29.7)	(38.2)	(2.1)	(1.7)	(9.5)	(2.70)	(3.7)
Total income of household (US$)	443.8	509.2	696.9	196.3	264.3	201.2	298.8	263.9	139.4	157.5
	(28.1)	(49.1)	(55.7)	30.0	(46.8)	(12.8)	(22.1)	(25.6)	(10.9)	(10.0)
Assets										
Own a car (%)	26.9	51.0	1.9	4.8						
Own land (%)	14.8	4.1	13.9	2.4						
Own house (%)	15.2	34.7	10.2	15.7						

and 33%, respectively, and between one third and one half of doctors in the regions outside Addis report receiving housing allowances (although we do not have data on the monetary value of these allowances). Indeed, significant shares of doctors working outside the Addis private sector report holding more than one job—from 23% in the Addis public sector, to 12% in Tigray. On the other hand, private-sector doctors in Addis supplement their (much higher) salaries by only 3%. Although 20% report holding more than one job, we expect that these multiple jobs are in some sense considered together to make up the worker's primary occupation, which accounts for the small amount of supplemental income. Finally, physician household incomes are higher in Addis than elsewhere.

The breakdown of physician and household incomes across regions is illustrated in Figure 1.5, and the corresponding data for nurses are presented in Figure 1.6. Interestingly, while household incomes of *private-sector* doctors in Addis trump those of households of doctors in the public sector and the outer regions, nurses who work in the *public* sector in Addis have higher household incomes than nurses in the private sector in Addis (despite their earning lower salaries than private-sector nurses in Addis). The opportunities to earn extra income outside of their primary jobs seem to be acutely attenuated for nurses.

We provide further statistical analysis of the differences between physician jobs in Addis Ababa and the regions in Table 1.8. This table confirms that differences in labor market outcomes between Addis and the regions do not merely reflect differences in observable characteristics of survey respondents. Controlling for experience levels and variables that predict the location of the worker's first job (separately for the lottery and non-lottery samples), the table presents estimates of labor market outcomes. We find that physicians currently working in Addis earn salaries that are between 60 and 85% higher, are between about 20 and 50% more likely to be specialized, and are considerably more content with various aspects of their work (especially those who are currently working in Addis and who initially participated in the lottery).[5]

In sum, these tables support the presumption that on average, a job in Addis Ababa is more attractive than one outside the capital. They first show that the overall quality of the facility faced by the average doctor in terms of observable inputs is similar across the regions, although patient-doctor ratios do favor Addis. Instead, as shown in the last table,

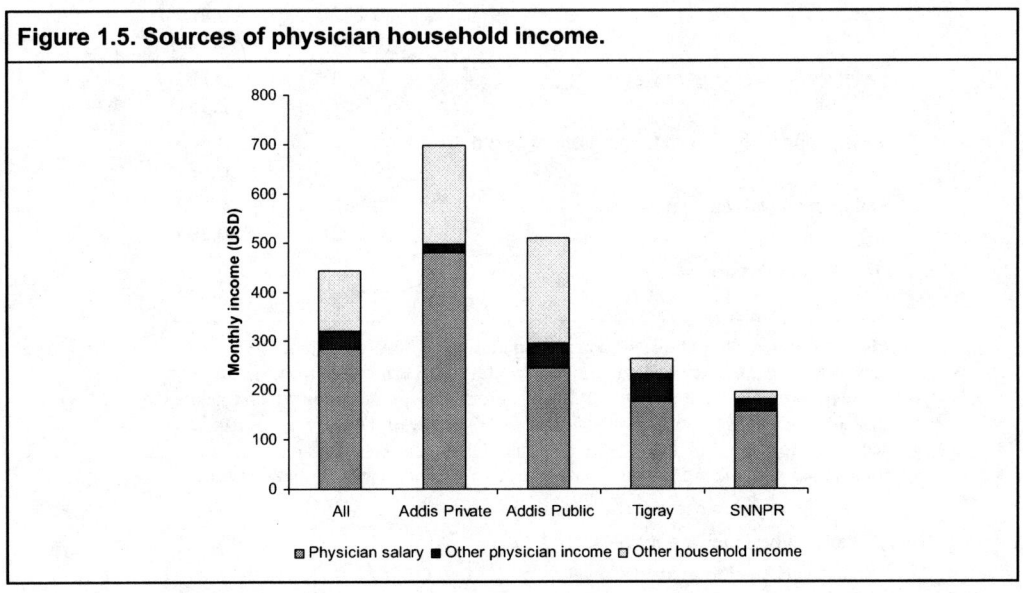

Figure 1.5. Sources of physician household income.

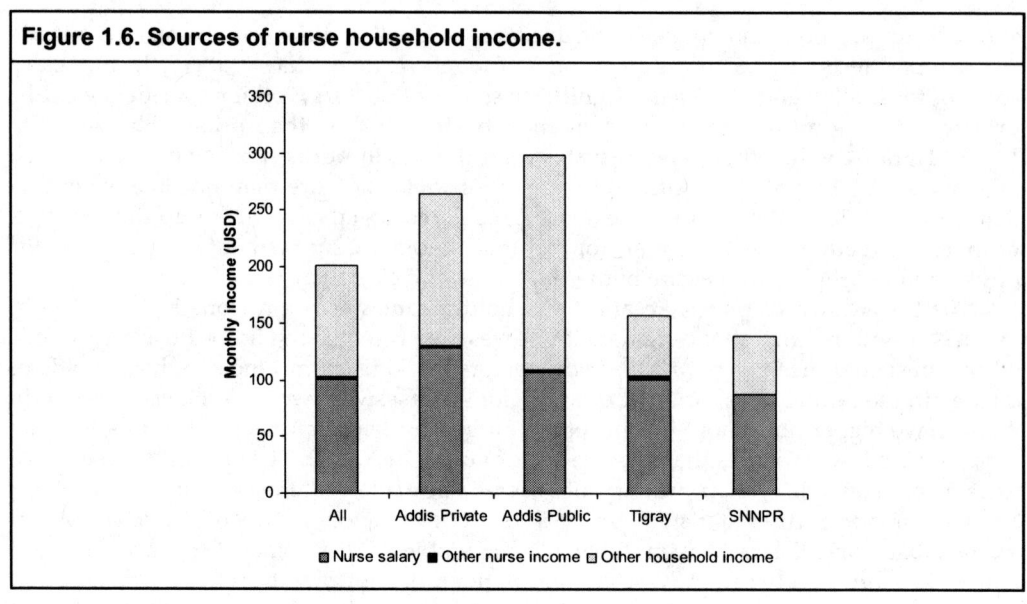

Figure 1.6. Sources of nurse household income.

Legend: ▨ Nurse salary ■ Other nurse income ▢ Other household income

Table 1.8. Impact of Currently Working in Addis on Physician Job Characteristics and Satisfaction

	Lottery	Market
Current salary (log)	0.815***	0.789***
	(0.144)	(0.167)
Current income (log)	0.728***	0.781***
	(0.177)	(0.156)
Doctor is specialized	0.232**	0.476***
	(0.104)	(0.112)
Satisfaction with current wage	0.925**	0.793
	(0.457)	(0.581)
Satisfaction with current training opportunities	−0.047	−0.465
	(0.313)	(0.421)
Satisfaction with current workload	0.769***	0.576
	(0.302)	(0.396)
Overall satisfaction with job	0.653*	0.827**
	(0.389)	(0.373)

Notes: Lottery includes those who participated in the lottery, while market includes those who did not. Each cell represents a separate OLS estimation (rows 1 and 2) or (ordered) probit estimation (rows 3–7) and reports the coefficient on a dummy variable indicating whether the current job is in Addis (1) or one of the two regions (0). The dependent variable is in the left-hand column. Other controls are: class rank, family connections with the profession, sponsor, sex, experience, siblings, and birth order.

*** Statistically significant at 1%-level

** Statistically significant at 5%-level

* Statistically significant at 10%-level

differences in labor market outcomes and satisfaction are more likely the principal reasons that physicians would prefer to work in Addis. Note too that non-lottery physicians currently working in Addis are significantly more content with their jobs overall than their non-lottery counterparts working in the rural regions, despite not being more content about their much higher salaries, their workload, and their training opportunities. This suggests that Addis Ababa is likely to have favorable characteristics not directly related to employment, but more related to what we might refer to as quality of life.

Analytic Results: The Performance of the Physician Labor Market

Next we explore two questions underlying the performance of the physician labor market in Ethiopia. The first asks what is the long-term impact of starting one's career in the rural areas. This is important because it can help us understand the costs associated with inducing labor supply to these regions. It is understandable that we might need to pay workers a premium to compensate them for the *flow* disutility and income loss they suffer while they are located outside the capital. But if there are long-term costs imposed on workers who spend time in rural areas, then recruits will additionally need to be compensated for the reduction in the *stock* of human capital they suffer as a result of living and working in remote areas. We use the nearly random nature of the lottery system for assigning jobs to new graduates, and other information, to identify this effect.

The second aspect of the labor market that we examine relates to the impact of the lottery itself on future labor market outcomes for physicians who take part in it. We find some evidence that suggests that the randomness of the allocation mechanism, although imperfect, and although possibly fair in some sense, induces an inefficiency in *future* physician labor markets. We suggest this is in fact because of the very (quasi-)randomness that characterises the lottery: random job assignments early on obfuscate information about workers that is useful to future employers, thereby potentially limiting the efficiency of the labor market later on. We find some evidence of this in wage dispersions among lottery participants and non-participants, and suggestions that attrition from the profession is higher among lottery participants.

The Labor Market Effects of Working in Rural Areas

Table 1.9 reports participation in the lottery and other labor market data for the physicians in our sample. Across the regions and the public and private sectors in

Table 1.9. Institutional Features of the Physician Labor Market

(%)	All	Addis		SNNPR	Tigray
		Public	Private		
Participated in the lottery	57.4	62.0	56.0	54.7	58.1
First job in Addis Ababa:					
of lottery participants	12.8	24.5	17.9	1.6	0.0
of non-participants	19.9	31.0	36.4	0	2.8
Medical training sponsored					
by federal government	71.4	67.7	80.0	70.1	59.3
Specialist training	27.4	40.4	38.0	6.8	19.8
Applied for official release					
from public sector	44.9	38.7	86.0	19.7	4.7
of whom, release granted	84.1	73.9	95.3	47.8	25.0

Addis, about 60% of respondents had participated in the lottery when being assigned their first job. Of those who participated in the lottery, 12.8% got their first position in Addis, while among those who did not participate in the lottery, the share who started their careers in Addis was 19.9%. If participation in the lottery was random, so that lottery participants were on average identical to those who chose not to participate in the lottery, and if job assignment under the lottery mechanism itself was random, then we could use the lottery to estimate the impact on future career development of getting a first job in Addis.

In fact, the data we collected reject both of these underlying assumptions. To start, lottery participants appear to be systematically different to non-participants: first, participants in the lottery tend to report having received lower grades in medical school; second they graduated less recently and were less likely to report that private health clinics were common when they started medical school; and third, they were more likely to have received federal government sponsorship for their training (as opposed to sponsorship from a regional government or from private or foreign sources). The regression results of one specification are presented in Table 1.10. This table also highlights the potential importance of the private sector in determining lottery participation. In the survey, we asked respondents whether private clinics were common when they started medical school, and we find that this variable reduces participation in the lottery.

In light of these results on lottery participation, we cannot easily extrapolate the labor market experiences of those who participated in the lottery to the rest of the population of physicians, as they differ on dimensions that could themselves affect career prospects.

Table 1.10. Predicting Participation in the Lottery

Predicting lottery participation	
2nd-ranked student	−0.081
	(0.098)
3rd-ranked student	0.234**
	(0.093)
Sponsor: private/foreign government	−0.447***
	(0.109)
Years experience	0.071***
	(0.015)
Years experience squared	−0.002***
	(0.000)
Birth order	−0.062**
	(0.027)
Number of siblings	0.037*
	(0.019)
Private clinics were common when starting medical school	−0.512***
	(0.151)
2nd-rank x private clinics were common when starting medical school	0.466***
	(0.053)
3rd-rank x private clinics were common when starting medical school	0.196
	(0.313)
Observations	216
Pseudo R-squared	0.2130

Notes: Probit model, dprobit coefficients reported. P-values: *** 1%, ** 5%, * 10%. Std errors corrected for clustering at facility level.

However, *within* the group of physicians who participated in the lottery, we can make some inferences about the effects of assignment to the rural areas, even though we have evidence that job assignment under the lottery was not truly random. We find that assignment to the rural areas under the lottery was more likely for males and for those who had recevied sponsorship from a regional government for medical school. Importantly, we do not find any correlation between family connections with the medical profession and lottery assignment—that is, while there is anecdotal evidence that the lottery is manipulated by certain people, our data do not reject the hypothesis that such manipulations are absent. Of course, a longer and more probing questionnaire might have uncovered other determinants of job assignment under the lottery, including the influence of friends and/or relatives in positions of authority.

The determinants of first job assignment amongst those who *did not* participate in the lottery are orthogonal to those of lottery participants. Among this group, we find that good performance in medical school predicts assignment to Addis, and that connection to the medical profession is also important, although in a subtle way: having parents in the health sector actually reduced the chance of getting a job in Addis for those not participating in the lottery, while having other relatives (uncles and/or aunts) increased it. Those variables that predict the location of lottery participants' first jobs—sex and sponsorship—are not significant in explaining where lottery non-participants get their first jobs. These results are presented in Table 1.11. The two columns labelled "I" include all right-hand-side variables, while the two labelled "II" include those that are significant in specification I (as well as the second dummy for private/foreign government sponsor for lottery participants). This highlights the very different determinants of the location of physicians' first jobs under the lottery and market.

Correcting for these correlations, and employing statistical matching techniques, we are able to estimate the impact of being assigned to Addis Ababa versus the rural areas on a number of dimensions of a physician's subsequent career development. Interestingly, for lottery participants, being assigned to Addis by the lottery is not a guarantee of long-term benefits. Those assigned to Addis rather than to one of the rural regions are no more likely to be working in Addis now, to have employment in the private sector, or to have significantly higher wages in their current employment, than those who were assigned to an outer region. Somewhat surprisingly, we find that lottery physicians assigned to Addis are significantly less likely than others to be specialized now (between 15% and 18%), so starting a career in the capital is not necessarily a ticket to specialization—if anything, the opposite appears to be true. In contrast, as shown in columns 3 and 4, both the OLS and NNM estimates indicate that market physicians with a first assignment in Addis are more likely to be specialized. One explanation for this difference is that Addis attracts high-ranking medical students through the market, with whom average-ranked lottery students must compete for specialist training.

Table 1.12 shows that, except for the specialization estimate, the estimates for market physicians are unclear. None of the other coefficients on being first assigned to Addis in the OLS estimates are significant, while all NNM estimates are very significant yet unclear. They suggest that physicians landing a job in Addis after medical school are significantly more likely to still be working there, and earn higher incomes, but are less likely to work in the private sector and less satisfied with their current job. We are reluctant to interpret these non-lottery findings, not only because of likely omitted variable bias, but because these NNM non-lottery findings are very sensitive to the matching variables.

In sum, these estimates suggest that in the long run there is a fair amount of mobility following the initial lottery assignments. Still, physicians assigned to Addis through the lottery may fare slightly better than those assigned to the rural area, as measured by their current job satisfaction. This is despite having lower levels of specialization than lottery physicians initially assigned to the rural regions. The bottom row of the table may be able

Table 1.11. Predicting Assignment to Addis Ababa in First Job after Medical School

	Predicting first job in Addis Ababa							
	Lottery				Market			
	I		II		I		II	
2nd-ranked student	0.078 (0.078)				−0.173 (0.114)	126	−0.209 (0.131)	126
3rd-ranked student	0.029 (0.100)				−0.297 (0.148)	*	−0.248 (0.122)	**
Parents health workers	−0.031 (0.083)				−0.341 (0.194)	*	−0.258 (0.118)	**
Other relatives health workers	0.046 (0.102)				0.259 (0.127)	**	0.300 (0.105)	***
Sponsor: regional authorities	−0.190 (0.055)	***	−0.146 (0.053)	***	0.022 (0.098)			
Sponsor: private/ foreign government	0.090 (0.107)		0.105 (0.103)		0.022 (0.161)			
Male (=1)	−0.232 (0.097)	**	−0.228 (0.087)	**	−0.127 (0.176)			
Years experience	0.011 (0.016)				−0.006 (0.019)			
Years experience squared	−0.001 (0.001)				0.000 (0.001)			
Order of birth	−0.011 (0.017)				0.034 (0.028)			
Number of siblings	0.022 (0.017)				−0.024 (0.031)			
Observations	122		122		85		85	
R-squared	0.1451		0.0971		0.2249		0.1915	

Notes: Linear probability model. P-values: *** 1%, ** 5%, * 10%.

Standard errors corrected for clustering at facility level.

to reconcile these findings. Physicians assigned to Addis are significantly more likely to be living now in the region they used to live in as adolescents, suggesting that despite lower specialization, they may benefit from non-employment-related compensating differences.

The Effects of Participating in the Lottery

Is the lottery an efficient and effective mechanism for allocating physician labor immediately after graduation? To answer this question, we ask whether using the lottery to allocate physicians to jobs early in their careers has any impact on the long-run workings of the labor market. In particular, we examine the effects of the lottery itself on future wages, the location of future jobs, and the provision of training. We can examine the impact of the lottery on these outcomes because we can compare the careers of physicians who participated in the lottery with the careers of those who did not, correcting for other differences betweeh the two groups when necessary.

Table 1.12. Estimates of the Long-Term Effects of Starting a Career in Addis Ababa

| | Effects of first job in Addis | | | |
| | Lottery participants | | Market participants | |
Dependent variable	(OLS)	(NNM)	(OLS)	(NNM)
Currently working in Addis	0.165	−0.109	0.046	0.421***
	(0.210)	(0.154)	(0.131)	(0.098)
Physician is specialized	−0.149**	−0.176***	0.195*	0.426***
	(0.065)	(0.040)	(0.097)	(0.143)
Currently working in private sector	0.164	−0.037	0.014	−0.627***
	(0.166)	(0.103)	(0.192)	(0.131)
Current salary (log)	0.161	−0.011	0.065	0.345**
	(0.170)	(0.091)	(0.186)	(0.155)
Overall satisfaction with current job	0.687	0.202	0.087	−3.132***
	(0.369)	(0.322)	(0.582)	(0.474)
Physician currently lives in the same	0.386***	0.433***	−0.123	−0.259***
region in which (s)he lived at age ten	(0.097)	(0.048)	(0.186)	(0.073)
Number observations	121	121	85	85

Notes: Each cell represents the estimate (or standard error) of the effect of having a first job in Addis on the dependent variable listed in the first column. Other controls included are class rank, connections to medical profession, medical school sponsor, sex, experience, birth order, and number of siblings. Physicians with less than two years experience are excluded.

*** Statistically significant at 1%-level

** Statistically significant at 5%-level

* Statistically significant at 10%-level

We find some evidence that the lottery system impedes the efficient working of the physician labor market, perhaps because it reduces the strength of the signal a physician's first job might provide to future employers. The idea is that future employers might use information about a physician's first job to learn about the physician's quality, but if the lottery *randomly* assigns graduates to their first jobs, these jobs provide no useful information to future employers about the underlying characeristics of workers. As we saw above, if a physician received a high rank at medical school—which we assume is an indicator of high underlying ability—he or she is more likely to get a first job in Addis, as long as he or she did not participate in the lottery. Having a first job in Addis is thus a signal of quality, but only for non-participants in the lottery. For lottery participants, a first job in Addis provides no information about underlying physician quality, and thus could lead to adverse selection in the physician labor market. As a consequence, high-quality phyisicians from the lottery will likely get paid less later in their careers than similar physicians who did not participate in the lottery. Also, high-quality lottery physicians will be more likely to drop out of the profession later on, as they find that they cannot command a salary commensurate with their skills.

Effects on Wages

If information on worker quality is publicly observable, then a physician's first job does not provide a useful signal to future employers. In our empirical analysis, we do allow for the possibility that working in Addis Ababa (either in a good facility or in a place with access to other colleagues and a richer learning environment) has a real, positive effect

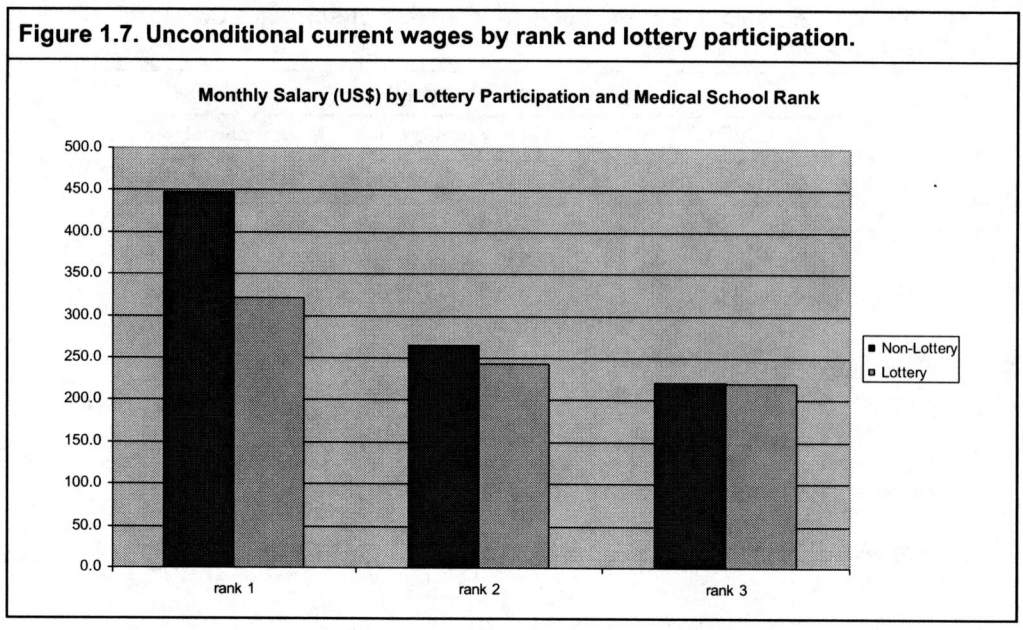

Figure 1.7. Unconditional current wages by rank and lottery participation.

Monthly Salary (US$) by Lottery Participation and Medical School Rank

on productivity. In this case, conditioning on class rank, future wages may be positively correlated with having a first job in Addis. However, the distribution of wages should be the same for both lottery participants and those who enter the market immediately after graduation. On the other hand, if the lottery obfuscates worker quality information, then we expect that the conditional wage distribution will be narrowed. Figure 1.7, which shows the unconditional wage distribution by rank separately for lottery and non-lottery physicians, provides suggestive evidence to this effect.

Consistent with the model, the graph shows that physicians who were third-ranked students earn virtually the same whether they were initially in the lottery or not. Among second-ranked students, non-lottery doctors earn slightly more, but not much. However, there is a large difference among first-ranked physicians, with non-lottery physicians earning 39% more on average. Table 1.13 explores this in a regression context, predicting log wages using interactions between class rank and lottery participation. Here, third rank is the left-out category to highlight the focus on first-rank dynamics.

Due to power limitations, we first force the impact of lottery participation on third-ranked physicians to be zero, consistent with Figure 1.7. Table 1.13 then uses separate dummies to allow wage levels of first- and second-ranked physicians to differ, but combines first and second rank in their interaction with lottery participation. The coefficients indicate that, compared with third-ranked physicians, second-ranked physicians earn 19% (0.187) more if they are outside the lottery but earn the same as third-ranked physicians inside the lottery (a combination of the direct effect and the interaction, 0.187 − 0.227); first-ranked physicians earn 48% (0.482) more outside the lottery, but only 26% more inside the lottery (a combination of the direct and effect and the interaction, 0.482 − 0.227).

Effects on Attrition from the Physician Labor Market

Wage compression among lottery participants may induce high-ability physicians who participated in the lottery to quit the profession. The data—illustrated in Figure 1.8—provide supportive, although not conclusive, evidence for this possibility. First, the time

Table 1.13. Effects of Lottery Participation on Future Wages

	Predicting Log Monthly Salary	
1st-ranked student	0.482	***
	(0.131)	
2nd-ranked student	0.187	126
	(0.118)	
1st- & 2nd-ranked student x	−0.227	*
lottery participation	(0.114)	
Experience	0.059	***
	(0.018)	
Experience squared (x 100)	−0.152	***
	(0.052)	
Sponsor: regional authorities	−0.289	*
	(0.151)	
Sponsor: private/foreign government	−0.120	
	(0.111)	
Birth order	0.072	***
	(0.026)	
Number of siblings	−0.025	
	(0.017)	
Number observations	205	

Notes: Physicians with less than two years experience excluded.

P-values: *** 1%, ** 5%, * 10%, ~15%.

Robust standard errors clustered at the facility level.

series of lottery participation show a drop not just among the latest 2006 cohort, which is consistent with anecdotal evidence that the lottery is unravelling,[6] but also among the oldest cohorts who graduated before 1993. Anecdotal evidence suggests that government enforcement of the lottery has been declining over time, so one would expect that lottery participation would have been highest among the oldest cohorts. If this were the case, then

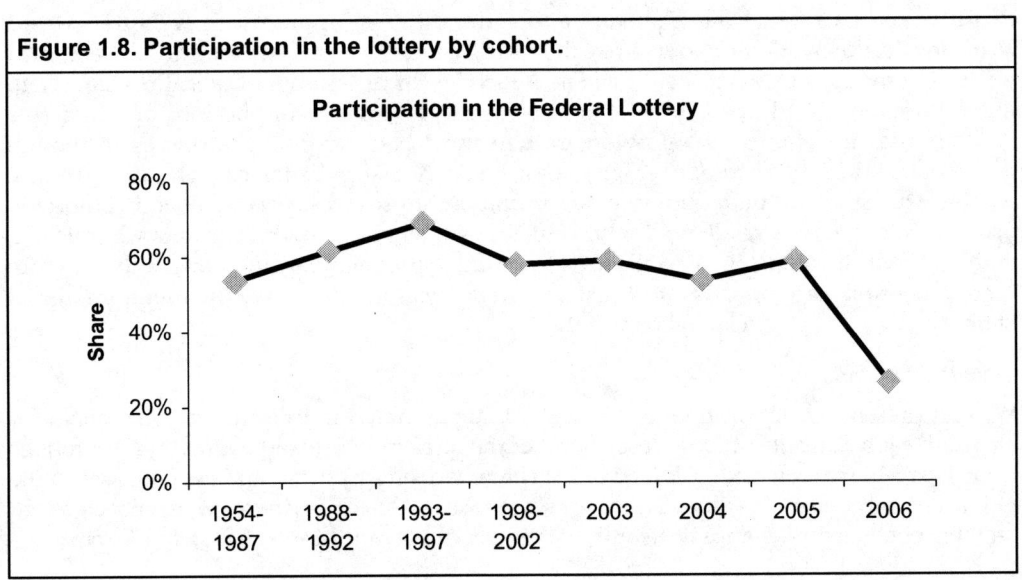

Figure 1.8. Participation in the lottery by cohort.

Table 1.14. Evidence of Labor Market Attrition by High-Ranked Lottery Participants

Predicting First Rank		
Lottery participant	0.149	
	(0.137)	
Lottery participant x experience	−0.018	*
	(0.010)	
Experience	0.033	*
	(0.017)	
Experience squared (x 100)	−0.074	126
	(0.047)	
Number observations	209	

Notes: Physicians with less than two years experience excluded.

P-values: * 10%, ~15%.

Robust standard errors clustered at the facility level.

differential attrition rates between lottery and non-lottery participants over time could have given rise to this pattern.

Table 1.14 explores in a regression context the extent to which high-ranked lottery participants have left the profession more than similar individuals who did not participate in the lottery. The dependent variable is a dummy for being first-ranked. The positive coefficient on experience (0.033) indicates that older cohorts are more likely to be first-ranked than younger cohorts, suggesting that over time first-ranked individuals have chosen not to enter the profession (in Ethiopia). On the other hand, the negative coefficient on the interaction between experience and lottery participation indicates that within older cohorts, lottery participants in our sample are less likely to be first-ranked than non-participants. This suggests that among high-ranked individuals, lottery participants have left the profession more than non-participants. This is consistent with the idea that the lottery has long-term impacts on the workings of the physician labor market.

Predictive Results: Rural Health Care—How Much Does It Cost?

Part II of our individual questionnaire adopted a different approach than Part I. Instead of asking health workers about what they did, what they earned, who they were, etc., we sought to find out what they *would do* if faced with certain hypothetical choices. With this information, we hoped to be able to estimate the relative importance of alternative job attributes and the trade-offs workers perceived between these attributes. Although the job attributes we focus on—higher pay, better housing, better equipment and more reliable drug supplies, better training opportunities, improved supervision, and authorized private-sector work—are all, no doubt, valued positively by workers, the data we collected in this part of the questionnaire allow us to estimate the relative valuations, and therefore represent a first step towards a full cost-benefit analysis of alternative interventions aimed at increasing rural physician labor supply.

Empirical Methodology

We first present a brief outline of the methodology employed to estimate preferences for alternative job attributes. A full description of the questionnaire and estimation techniques is provided in Hanson and Jack (2008). We characterized physician and nursing jobs in the public sector by discrete values of each of six attributes. These attributes were chosen based on their perceived relevance to health worker decisions in Ethiopia, following discussions

Table 1.15. Job Attributes and Levels

	Doctors	
	Attribute	**Possible levels**
X^1	Location	Addis Ababa vs. Regional Capital
X^2	Net Monthly Pay (*Base* = 2,500)	$1 \times Base$; $1.5 \times Base$; $2 \times Base$
X^3	Housing	None, Basic, Superior
X^4	Equipment and Drugs	Inadequate vs. Improved
X^5	Time Commitment	2 years vs. 1 year
X^6	Private Sector	Yes vs. No
	Nurses	
	Attribute	**Possible levels**
X^1	Location	City vs. Rural
X^2	Net Monthly Pay (*Base* = 1,250)	*Base*; $1.5 \times Base$; $2 \times Base$
X^3	Housing	None, Basic, Superior
X^4	Equipment and Drugs	Inadequate vs. Improved
X^5	Time Commitment	2 years vs. 1 year
X^6	Supervision	High vs. Low

with officials from the Federal Ministry of Health and the heads of regional health bureaus in Addis Ababa, Mekele (the capital of Tigray), and Awasa (the capital of the SNNPR). The attributes chosen are shown in Table 1.15.

The attribute *values* or *levels* were chosen both to be realistic and to provide a wide enough range of variation to enable predictions about relatively large policy to be made. The values of the location attribute differed for doctors and nurses. In practice, very few doctors work outside towns, so for them we allowed the location attribute to be either "Addis Ababa" or "Regional Capital." For nurses, however, this attribute took on the values "City" and "Rural." At the time of the study, public-sector health workers were paid on the basis of a pay scale based on experience, qualifications, etc. We used the (unweighted) average monthly salary from these scales to determine a "base" salary for doctors and nurses separately, and let the pay attribute take on values each to 1, 1.5, and 2 times this value. The third (housing), fourth (equipment and drugs), and fifth (time[7]) attributes in Table 1.15 took on the same values for doctors and nurses. For doctors, the final attribute was permission to work in the private sector (taking the values "yes" and "no"). Since opportunities for providing nursing services outside regular hours are limited, the opportunity to work in the private sector is of limited use for nurses. However, experience from other countries has suggested that active and supportive supervision is an important job attribute for these health workers. This is the sixth attribute we included for nurses.

Our questionnaire presented individuals with a series of 15 pairs of jobs, listed in Table 1.16, and asked them to choose the one they preferred from each pair.[8] We presented these choices in a variety of different formats to ensure that fatigue and/or lack of interest did not affect respondents' answers.

The data we collect allow us to estimate the average rates at which respondents trade off one attribute against another. In particular, when one of the attributes is pay, we can speak of the marginal monetary valuation of an attribute. In addition, we can use the data to ask what impact a given policy intervention—such as providing basic housing in rural

Table 1.16. The Constant Job, Job 1, and the 15 Comparator Jobs

	Location	Pay	Housing	Equipment and drugs	Payback time	Private sector/ Supervision
Job 1	Addis	1.5	Basic	Inadequate	1	Yes/High
Job 2	Addis	1.5	Superior	Inadequate	2	Yes/High
Job 3	Rural	1	Superior	Improved	2	Yes/High
Job 4	Rural	1	Basic	Improved	1	Yes/High
Job 5	Addis	1	None	Improved	1	Yes/High
Job 6	Rural	1.5	None	Improved	2	No/Low
Job 7	Rural	1.5	None	Improved	1	No/Low
Job 8	Addis	1	None	Inadequate	2	No/Low
Job 9	Rural	2	None	Inadequate	2	Yes/High
Job 10	Addis	2	Superior	Improved	1	No/Low
Job 11	Rural	1	Superior	Inadequate	1	No/Low
Job 12	Addis	1	None	Improved	2	Yes/High
Job 13	Rural	1	Basic	Inadequate	2	No/Low
Job 14	Addis	2	Basic	Improved	2	No/Low
Job 15	Rural	2	Basic	Inadequate	1	No/Low
Job 16	Addis	1	Basic	Inadequate	1	Yes/High

areas—will have on the share of workers willing to accept jobs there, and we can calculate the rural wage bonus that would have an equivalent effect on labor supply. This method of converting in-kind interventions into wage equivalents allows us to compare interventions in a more meaningful way. Finally, we estimate the impact of wage bonuses *and* selected in-kind interventions on labor supply responses.

Valuing Job Attributes

Table 1.17 reports average (marginal) valuations of each of the non-wage job attributes, measured as a percentage of the baseline public sector salary (2,500 Birr, or $275, per month for doctors; 1,250 Birr, or $140, per month for nurses). These figures were estimated.

These results suggest that on average, the extra value of a job in Addis relative to one in a regional city for doctors amounts to about one quarter (27%) of the base public sector physician salary; the value of improved housing is about one third (32%); the value of equipment is about one quarter (26%); and the value of reduced time commitment is about

Table 1.17. The Direct-Effects Model, for Doctors and Nurses

	Value as % of base salary	
Variable	Doctors	Nurses
Location	26.8%	72.1%
Improved Housing	32.4%	46.9%
Adequate Equipment and Drugs	26.4%	49.9%
Payback Time	18.2%	11.6%
Private sector/Supervision	48.0%	32.6%

one fifth (18%). However, the most highly prized attribute for doctors is the ability to work in the private sector, which has a value of about half (48%) the base salary.

For nurses the most valuable job attribute is location. Indeed, location appears to be valued more by nurses than by doctors, especially when the value is measured as a share of the base salary. This partly reflects the fact that "location" means something different in the questions nurses were presented with than it does for doctors—switching a job from a rural area, which in principle can be very remote, to a regional capital, increases its value by 72% of the base public sector nurse's salary. (The other factor is, of course, the fact that the base nurse salary is only half the base doctor salary.) The least valued attribute for nurses appears to be payback time, as it is for doctors—having to pay back an extra year after receiving training is equivalent to a pay cut of about 12% of base salary. Improved supervision is valued, but not as highly as the other non-time attributes.

The valuations reported in Table 1.17 reflect averages across different types of health workers, as characterized by age, sex, marital status, number of children, and current location. By including these individual characteristics in the empirical specification, we can examine the extent to which job attribute valuations vary across individuals in predictable ways.[9]

We find, for example, that married doctors value a job in Addis twice as highly as single doctors (38% versus 19% of base salary). In contrast, married nurses value urban work, and housing, *less* than single nurses. We do not know why marriage should affect nurses' valuations differently than those of doctors. One difference is, of course, that "location" means something different in our estimation of the preferences of nurses and doctors.[10]

The impact of children seems perhaps surprisingly small, particularly the impact of the first child: Doctors with one child value an Addis job (presumably with better schools, etc.) just 2 percentage points of base salary more than doctors without children (30.6% versus 28.6%). For nurses, the impact of children seems somewhat larger than it is for doctors (in terms of the percentage of base salary), but again, having children does not seem to be an especially impenetrable barrier to rural work. The value of an urban job over a rural job is 60% of base salary for childless nurses, and 66% for those with one child. Thus, urban jobs are highly valued—but not particularly so for nurses with children.

Can In-Kind Incentives Significantly Increase Rural Labor Supply?

A useful way to interpret our estimated valuations is to use them to estimate the impacts of changes in job attributes on the probability that an individual will accept a job in a rural area over a job in Addis Ababa (for doctors) or in a regional capital (for nurses). Holding public-sector wages constant (i.e., without introducing wage bonuses), we calculate the change in the estimated probability of an individual accepting a rural job when one non-wage attribute is improved. The results of this exercise are reported in Table 1.18. Our point estimates indicate, for example, that about 7.5% of doctors would be willing to take a rural job over a job in Addis under prevailing conditions, if they had the choice.[11] Providing incentives in the form of superior housing increases the chance of accepting a rural job to more than one in four, while provision of basic housing, and training incentives (measured by a reduction in time commitment to one year) have relatively small effects, each increasing the likelihood from 7.5% to about 11%. The effect of improving the availability of equipment is in the middle of the range, increasing the probability of choosing a rural job to 17%. (We do not calculate the predicted labor supply increase in rural areas associated with permitting private sector work, since such work is relatively scarce outside of Addis Ababa.)

For nurses, the non-wage attribute with the single biggest impact on the share of workers willing to take a rural job is the provision of adequate equipment. At baseline levels, only 4.4% of nurses would choose a rural job over a city job, but this jumps to 20% if they can be guaranteed adequate levels of equipment. The provision of basic housing, reducing payback time, and providing better supervision have substantially smaller effects on the probability of choosing a rural job, increasing it to levels in the range of 5–8%.

Table 1.18. Impact of Non-Wage Attribute Improvement on Probability of Accepting a Rural Job, for Doctors

	Doctors			Nurses		
	p	95% CI	Increase	*p*	95% CI	Increase
Baseline	0.074	(0.029, 0.122)	—	0.046	(0.034, 0.058)	—
Basic housing	0.109	(0.046, 0.173)	47%	0.097	(0.080, 0.115)	112%
Superior housing	0.269	(0.137, 0.400)	262%	0.192	(0.152, 0.233)	319%
Equipment	0.167	(0.105, 0.229)	125%	0.198	(0.165, 0.231)	332%
Payback time	0.114	(0.047, 0.180)	53%	0.056	(0.041, 0.072)	22%
Equip & housing	0.226	(0.144, 0.308)	204%	0.323	(0.284, 0.362)	605%
Supervision	—	—	—	0.075	(0.055, 0.095)	64%

Wage Equivalents

Knowing that superior housing more than triples the willing supply of physician labor to rural areas is not particularly useful unless the cost of such a policy is known. Even if such cost information were available, policymakers would be advised to compare the costs with other policy interventions that had similar labor supply effects. While we do not have cost information on the in-kind interventions we examine in this research, we are able to estimate the wage bonuses that would have equivalent effects. Table 1.19 reports these wage equivalents (as percentages of the base salary) for doctors and nurses, and for men and women separately. Interestingly, while the point estimates of wage equivalents for most attributes tend to be higher for women, the difference is rarely statistically significantly. Figure 1.9 illustrates this by placing 95% confidence intervals around the estimated wage equivalents for each policy, by sex.

Combining Financial and In-Kind Incentives

Finally, we investigate the impact of increases in rural pay *and* improvements in other job attributes on health worker labor supply. The results, for doctors and nurses respectively, are presented graphically in Figures 1.10 and 1.11, respectively. For doctors, doubling pay while keeping other attributes constant increases the probability of accepting a rural job from 7% to 57%. Alternatively, to induce half of doctors to locate in rural areas under current conditions, a rural bonus of approximately 89% (2,225 Birr) is required. Providing basic housing does not affect the impact of wages to a large extent, probably because most doctors

Table 1.19. Wage Equivalents of Attribute Improvements, by Sex, for Doctors and Nurses

	Doctors		Nurses	
	Male	Female	Male	Female
Basic housing	11.7	12.3	44.1	53.7
Superior housing	45.2	47.3	92.6	112.7
Equipment and drug	24.6	35.7	57.4	69.9
Payback time	14.1	7.1	8.0	9.8
Equipment & housing	36.2	48.0	101.5	123.6
Supervision	—	—	31.3	38.2

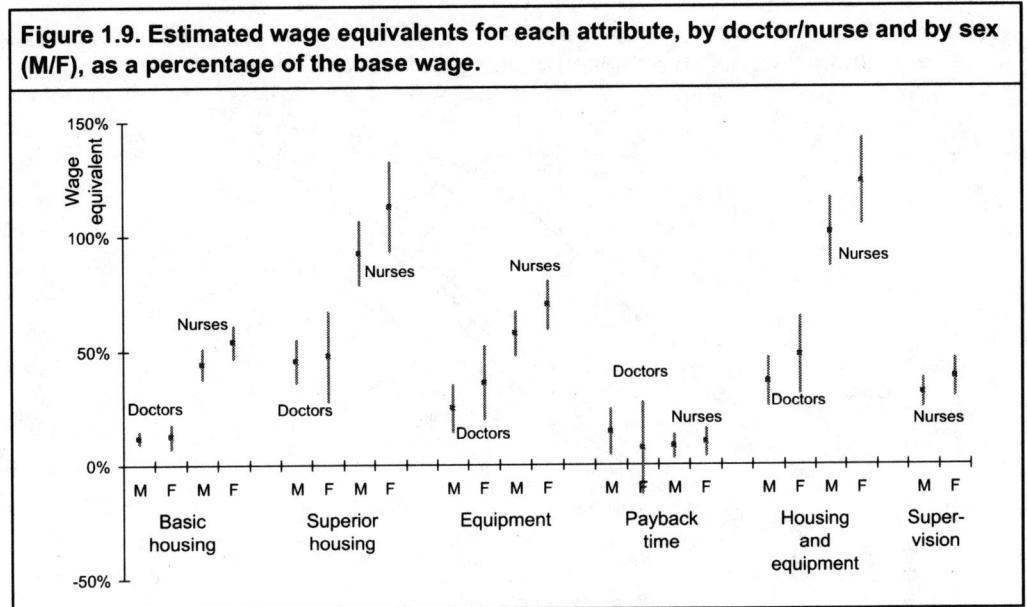

Figure 1.9. Estimated wage equivalents for each attribute, by doctor/nurse and by sex (M/F), as a percentage of the base wage.

already have at least basic housing. On the other hand, providing superior housing means that doubling wages increases the probability of accepting a rural job from 27% to 84%.

Our results suggest that nurses are much less responsive to proportionate wage bonuses than doctors—a doubling of pay increases the probability of accepting a rural job from 4% to only 27%, and inducing half of the nursing workforce to locate in rural areas would require a wage bonus of about 155% of the base salary. This bonus amounts to 1,937 Birr, and is only marginally smaller than that needed to induce a similar proportion of doctors to take jobs in rural areas. The impact of adequate equipment, both on willingness

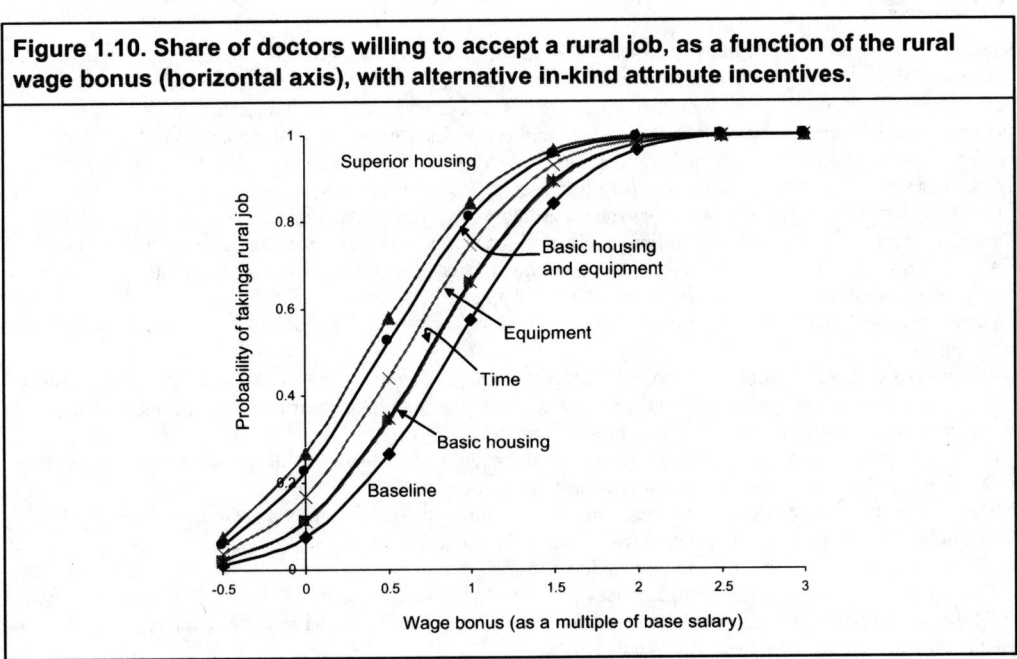

Figure 1.10. Share of doctors willing to accept a rural job, as a function of the rural wage bonus (horizontal axis), with alternative in-kind attribute incentives.

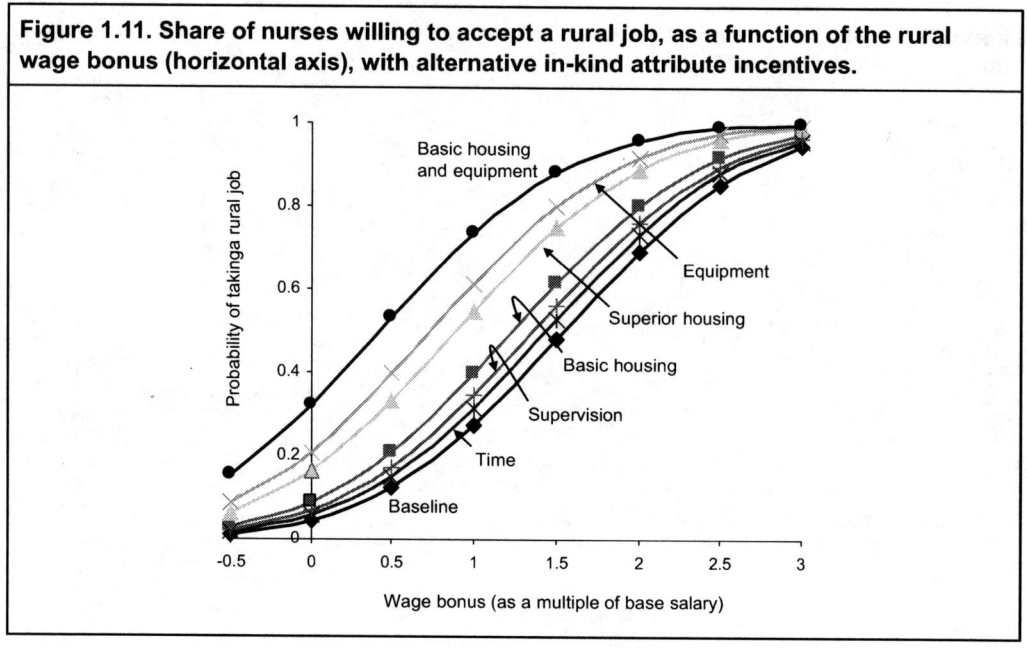

Figure 1.11. Share of nurses willing to accept a rural job, as a function of the rural wage bonus (horizontal axis), with alternative in-kind attribute incentives.

of nurses to take a rural job in itself and on the impact of higher pay on such willingness, is of particular interest, especially since this attribute does not reflect personal consumption as such. Indeed, the impact of equipment is not only greater than that of basic housing; it exceeds that of *superior* housing also. By itself, adequate equipment increases the likelihood of accepting a rural job from 4% to 21%; when coupled with a doubling of rural pay, this probability increases to 61%.

Notes

[1] The maximum number of health workers assigned to each region is decided before October by a three-person committee at the Ministry of Health, on the basis of the official requests for health workers sent by each region. An exception in the lottery system has been recently introduced with respect to the assignment to posts in the newest regions of Benishangul, Hafar, Somali, and Gambella. Before the lottery takes place, each health worker is asked whether he or she would be willing to work in any of these new regions. If the answer is negative, as in the majority of cases, the corresponding posts are added to the lottery.

[2] Other regions, such as Oromia (which surrounds Addis Ababa) and Amhara (which is immediately north of Oromia) are larger (with 26 and 19 million residents respectively) and less remote, at least in terms of direct distance measures, but we have no reason to expect this to have introduced systematic biases in our estimates.

[3] The complete survey instrument can be found in the Appendix.

[4] There are 77 such facilities in our survey, out of a total of 97. Twenty of the facilities visited are not staffed by a physician.

[5] Job satisfaction are self-reported answers (5 categories) ranging from "Not at all satisfied" to "Very satisfied."

[6] We are unable to identify whether this change reflects a real drop in lottery participation, delayed attrition from the health sector by non-participants, or a combination of both.

[7] Time refers to the number of years that an individual is required to work at an institution per year of further training sponsored by that institution, after the training is completed.

[8] With six attributes, each with two or three values, the number of possible job pairs is much larger (20,592). The number of choices used is consistent with practice in the health economics literature.

[9] See Hanson and Jack (2008) for a more detailed discussion.

[10] Perhaps it is more important for single nurses to be in a city "marriage market" than it is for single doctors.

[11] Of course, demand-side constraints mean that most health workers do not have much of a choice; they cannot all work for the public sector in Addis Ababa.

Bibliography

Anand, Sudhir and Barnighausen, Till (2004): "Human Resources and Health Outcomes: Cross-Country Econometric Study." *Lancet* 364 (9445):1603–9.

Chomitz, Kenneth, Gunawan Setiadi, Azrul Azwar, Nusye Ismail, and Widiyarti (1998): "What Do Doctors Want? Developing Incentives for Doctors to Serve in Indonesia's Rural and Remote Areas," World Bank Policy Research Working Paper 1888, World Bank, Washington DC.

De Laat, Joost, and William Jack (2008): "Adverse Selection and Career Outcomes in the Ethiopian Physician Labor Market," mimeo.

Hanson, Kara, and William Jack (2008): "Health Worker Preferences for Job Attributes in Ethiopia: Results from a Discrete Choice Experiment," mimeo.

Hole, A.R. (2007): "A Comparison of Approaches to Estimating Confidence Intervals for Willingness to Pay Measures," *Health Economics* 16(8): 827–40.

Huber, J., and K. Zwerina (1996): "The Importance of Utility Balance in Efficient Choice Designs." *Journal of Marketing Research* 33: 307–17.

Joint Learning Initiative (2004). *Human Resources for Health: Overcoming the Crisis.* Boston, MA: Joint Learning Initiative.

Ministry of Health, Government of Ethiopia (2005): statistical tables.

Mangham, L., and K. Hanson (2007): "Eliciting the Employment Preferences of Public Sector Nurses: Results from a Discrete Choice Experiment in Malawi," unpublished mimeo.

Penn-Kekana, L., D. Blaauw, K.S. Tint, D. Monareng, J. Chege (2005): "Nursing Staff Dynamics and Implications for Maternal Health Provision in Public Health Facilities in the Context of HIV/AIDS." Johannesburg: Centre for Health Policy, University of the Witswatersrand.

Ryan, M., and K. Gerard (2003): "Using Discrete Choice Experiments in Health Economics: Moving Forward." In A. Scott, A. Maynard, and R. Elliott R, eds. *Advances in Health Economics.* New York: John Wiley and Sons.

Ryan, M., and K. Gerard (2003): "Using Discrete Choice Experiments to Value Health Care Programmes: Current Practice and Future Research Reflections." *Applied Health Economics and Health Policy,* 2(1): 55–64.

Scott, A. (2001): "Eliciting GPs' Preferences for Pecuniary and Non-pecuniary Job Characteristics." *Journal of Health Economics* 20: 329–47.

Serneels, Pieter, José García-Montalvo, Magnus Lindelow, and Abigail Barr (2005): "For Public Service or for Money: Understanding Geographical Imbalances in the Health Workforce." World Bank Policy Research Working Paper 3686, World Bank, Washington DC.

WHO (2006): *World Health Report 2006: Working Together for Health.* Geneva: World Health Organization.

Wilbulpolprasert, S., and P. Pengpaibon (2003): "Integrated Strategies to Tackle the Inequitable Distribution of Doctors in Thailand: Four Decades of Experience." *Human Resources for Health,* 1: 12.

CHAPTER 2

Long-Term Career Dynamics

Joost de Laat and William Jack

Introduction

Ethiopia faces acute challenges in reaching all of the Millenium Development Goals, including the three goals relating to health—to reduce child mortality, improve maternal health, and combat HIV/AIDS, malaria, and other diseases. This paper assesses one factor that will be important in moving toward these goals: the performance of the physician labor market.

There is, on average, about one physician for every 30,000 people in Ethiopia (Ministry of Health, 2005), three times the ratio recommended by the WHO. Rural and remote areas of the country are particularly underserved, and by some estimates up to half of the physicians work in the capital, Addis Ababa, home to about 5% of the population. Increasing labor supply in rural areas can be effected either by fiat or with financial and other incentives. The Ethiopian government has traditionally relied on the first approach, through the operation of a lottery-based clearinghouse for the assignment of new medical school graduates to their first postings.

In this paper we use recently collected data from a survey of physicians to address two basic questions about the physician labor market. First, what are the long-term effects of rural assignment on a health worker's career prospects? And second, how does the lottery system affect the subsequent efficiency of the physician labor market? In addressing each of these questions, we use data both on physicians who participated in the lottery system and on those who chose to enter the market directly.

There are three potential selection nodes in the allocation of newly graduated physicians to jobs.[1] First, although the lottery mechanism is officially mandatory, only about 60% of our sample participated, suggesting an element of choice. Second, for those who enter the lottery, job assignment could exhibit some non-randomness, due either to specific aspects of the allocation mechanism or to less formal bargaining and lobbying by some graduates. And third, for those who opt out of the lottery mechanism, assignment is potentially influenced by the preferences on both the demand and supply sides of the market. Our data suggest that the determinants of job assignment differ significantly between the second and third nodes. In particular, assignment under the lottery is close to random.

We use matching and standard regression techniques to identify the career impact of assignment to the rural areas, both among lottery participants and across all doctors. We find that lottery participants initially assigned to Addis are no more likely to be (a) currently working in Addis, (b) working in the private sector, or (c) earning higher salaries than those whose first job was outside the capital. Indeed, Addis assignment early on in the career *reduces* physician specialization rates, while increasing current job satisfaction and the likelihood that physicians are currently working in the their home regions.

Our evidence regarding the impact of assignment to Addis has interesting parallels in the recent education literature. Cullen et al. (2006) find that prospective high school students winning a lottery that gives them the option to attend a high-performing school in Chicago *do not* seem to benefit. In fact, they demonstrate that students who, *ex ante*, stand to gain the most in terms of peer quality in practice appear to be hurt by winning the lottery, at least in terms of academic outcomes. For example, they are more likely to drop out.

In our data, lottery physicians assigned to Addis find themselves among some of the relatively high-ability physicians who opted out of the lottery and found employment in Addis. As in the Chicago education study, this peer effect seems also to have negative consequences, perhaps because the " lucky winners" must compete against higher-ability doctors for specialist training opportunities, etc. As Cullen et al. point out, their findings are consistent with the literature on the importance of mismatch (e.g., Light and Strayer [2000]) and of one's relative position (e.g., Kaufman and Rosenbaum [1992]).

To examine the efficiency effects of the lottery system, we propose a model of adverse selection in the physician labor market. The idea is that some jobs are more desirable than others, and that under a market-based mechanism these jobs go to better-quality doctors. Initial job assignment then provides useful information to future employers regarding worker productivity. On the other hand, if jobs are initially allocated randomly, then future employers learn little about an individual's inherent ability from the location of this first job. For this group of workers, the labor market is subject to adverse selection, with relatively high-quality workers opting out of the profession.

We develop empirically testable implications of this theory and assess them using our newly collected dataset. The short-run implications of the model, pertaining to the allocation of new graduates, are broadly supported by the data: we find that first, the market allocates new graduates to jobs based at least in part on their ability and locational preferences. In contrast, these variables do not predict the initial assignment across regions for lottery participants. In light of this, higher-ability graduates tend to opt out of the lottery. The data also indicate that recent growth of demand for private-sector physicians is associated with falling lottery participation. And finally, the pattern of job satisfaction expressed among lottery participants across ability levels reflects the random nature of the lottery assignment: physicians assigned by the lottery to Addis are on average more satisfied with their first assignment.

Second, the data broadly support the long-term predictions of the model regarding the efficiency of the physician labor market. For example, we observe wage compression in the market for physicians who participated in the lottery: high-ability physicians who participated in the lottery earn significantly less (16%) than those who did not, while lottery participation does not significantly affect the future wages of lower-ability doctors. Similarly, access to future training opportunities appears to be attenuated for high-ability lottery participants relative to similar physicians who opted out of the lottery, while there is little such difference for lower-ability graduates. Finally, in light of these dynamics, we find evidence of higher rates of attrition among high-ability physicians who took part in the lottery than for those who did not. These results suggest that the lottery allocation obscures information about physician quality and may lead to adverse selection.

Ethiopia's Market for Physician Labor

The number of health workers working in Ethiopia is difficult to estimate. The Ministry of Health (2005) reports that in 2005 there were a total of 2,543 physicians, of which 444 (17%) operated in the private sector, 578 (23%) in the NGO sector, and 354 (14%) in other government organizations (such as the military). Of the 1,077 physicians classified as working for the public sector, 20%, or about 215, were located in Addis Ababa.

In recent years, there has been rapid growth in the private health care sector, but the vast majority of this growth has occurred in Addis Ababa. In fact, according to survey data we collected in 2006 on physicians in Ethiopia, 380 out of an estimated 597 physicians working in Addis (or 64%) currently work as physicians outside the public sector, the vast majority in the private sector, earning salaries that are double those in the public sector in Addis and triple those in the public sector outside Addis. In one of the two other regions covered by the survey, the SNNPR, about 10% of physicians are estimated to be working outside the public sector (including NGOs). In the second region, Tigray, virtually all doctors are estimated to work in the public sector.

As suggested by these statistics and confirmed through discussions with health workers themselves, attracting physicians to remote areas is a particular challenge. The problem of rural employment has grown even more acute as opportunities to work abroad expand, partly due to active recruitment efforts of other countries. For example, Clemens and Pettersson (2007) find that 30% of all practicing Ethiopian physicians work abroad.

The primary vehicle by which the supply of rural health workers is maintained is a national clearinghouse. Each year a national lottery is announced through the media in September. Health workers who graduated in the previous June and July, as well as doctors who have completed their internships, are invited to go to the Ministry of Health, starting in October, to participate in the lottery.

Under the lottery, which is officially mandatory, although in practice optional, a participant is randomly assigned to one of the twelve regions of the country. Job assignments at the regional level are administrated by the relevant regional health bureau (World Bank, 2006). Assigned workers are usually expected to serve a fixed number of years before being "released" and permitted to apply for other positions.[2]

National clearinghouses for entry-level physicians are also common in other countries. For example, in the United States, the market for almost all entry-level positions (called residencies) for new doctors is mediated by a clearinghouse called the National Resident Matching Program (NRMP). Applicants and employers submit rank-order lists representing their preferences, which are then used by the clearinghouse to centrally determine a match between applicants and employers (Niederle and Roth, 2007; Roth, 2008). Unlike the NRMP, the Ethiopian lottery system does not seek to explicitly match employer and physician preferences—at least not with respect to the regional location of job assignments.

While the lottery is still officially in place, during the past five years Ethiopia has embarked on a radical decentralization program across all areas of the public sector, with much of the responsibility for service delivery being devolved to lower levels of government. Regional competition for health workers, and the burgeoning private market, have arguably strengthened the incentives for certain new graduates to bypass the lottery and try their luck in the marketplace.

A Model of the Physician Labor Market

Motivation of the Model

In our pre-survey discussions with health workers, a number of potential benefits associated with working in Addis were identified, including higher wages and superior work and non-work amenities. Reflecting these observations, we assume that wage differentials in the entry-level physician labor market do not exactly offset the different costs and non-pecuniary benefits of working in different parts of the country. The resulting geographic imbalance of demand and supply in the physician labor market means jobs must be rationed by non-price mechanisms. The lottery and the market employ potentially different rationing systems, with different allocative properties.

This raises the question of whether a lottery is a good way to assign graduating physicians to jobs. On the one hand, random allocation is sometimes defended on the basis that it is fair, although this is only true in an *ex ante* sense.[3] On the other hand, economic theory suggests at least two reasons that a lottery might impact negatively on the workings of the labor market. First, in the short run, if there are important efficiency gains from matching individuals to jobs, then a truly random allocation will be inefficient, compared with an allocation mechanism that explicitly reflects preferences and costs, such as an idealized market.

Second, in the long run, using a lottery to allocate labor could obfuscate important information about health workers that is relevant to future employment decisions. For example, suppose there are important matching efficiencies in the market for graduating physicians. Among lottery participants, realized productivity in the first job (as revealed, for example, through letters of recommendation) may be a poor indicator of underlying potential productivity in a second assignment. Under a market mechanism, on the other hand, we might expect "good" graduates (those who were highly ranked in medical school) to be more likely to be matched to "good" jobs. Even if underlying ability is unobservable later in a physician's career, employers can use information about his or her first job as an indicator of quality in making their recruitment decisions. In particular, because jobs in Addis are rationed, we can use job location as such an indicator.

Assuming lottery participation itself is observable, the physician labor market will bifurcate into two sub-markets. In the lottery market, employers lack verifiable information on physician quality, which may lead to adverse selection. The effects could include compression in training opportunities and wages, and the departure of high-quality physicians from the market (either to other careers, or to migration). The non-lottery market, on the other hand, in which employers have a more informative signal of physician quality, might be expected to operate more efficiently.

These observations suggest that the labor market outcomes of lottery participants and non-participants may differ in systematic ways across different types of physicians. In pre-survey interviews, health officials linked recent expansion of the private sector with a downward trend in lottery participation. In light of this, we model lottery participation incentives as a function of expected search costs in the market, under the assumption that the growth of the private sector has reduced these costs.

We formalize the intuition above in the model below, and then test the implications on our dataset. Because we have detailed information on both lottery and non-lottery physicians, including details of their medical school performance, and their first and current assignments, we are able to investigate both the allocation mechanisms themselves and whether there is evidence of adverse selection among lottery physicians.

Adverse Selection in the Physician Labor Market

We propose a model in which there are two types of physicians—type L with low ability, and type H with high ability. The share of L-type physicians in the population is σ. There are also two types of "first" jobs—a first job in Addis, and a first job outside Addis. Physicians first choose whether to enter the lottery. If a physician stays out of the lottery, he suffers a random utility cost ε, which has distribution $G(\varepsilon)$. This disutility cost can be thought of as a search cost that the individual expects to incur in the labor market outside the lottery, or as an unknown cost imposed by the government, since lottery participation is officially mandatory.[4]

If a physician enters the lottery, he is randomly assigned to a first job by the government. With probability ρ he gets a job in Addis, and with probability $1 - \rho$ his first job is in a rural area. If he does not enter the lottery, he is assigned to a job by the market. We make the extreme assumption that the market assigns type H physicians to Addis and type L physicians outside Addis—effectively the market observes and rewards ability. We assume that all type L physicians enter the lottery, along with a fraction η of type H physicians. The assumption about type L physicians will be shown below to be correct in equilibrium, and the value of η will be calculated. Thus the share of the population of all physicians who participate in the lottery is

$$n^{Lott} = \underbrace{\sigma}_{L-types} + \underbrace{(1-\sigma)\eta}_{H-types}$$

There are $n^M \equiv (1-\sigma)(1-\eta)$ type H physicians who don't participate in the lottery and enter the market directly. The evolution of the labor market is shown in Figure 2.1.

After physicians have completed their first assignments, they all search for work, either in the profession (now through the market) or outside. By now, a physician's ability is known only by him, but the location of his first job is public information. For physicians who did not participate in the lottery, the market can use the location of the first as a perfect signal of ability, and reward it accordingly. Physicians who were not in the lottery receive a wage equal to their productivity: π_H for type H physicians, and $\pi_L < \pi_H$ for type L physicians. (In equilibrium all type L physicians are in the lottery.) For physicians who were in the lottery, the market must offer a constant wage. We assume that this is equal to the average productivity *of physicians who accept a job at that wage, $\bar{\pi}$.*

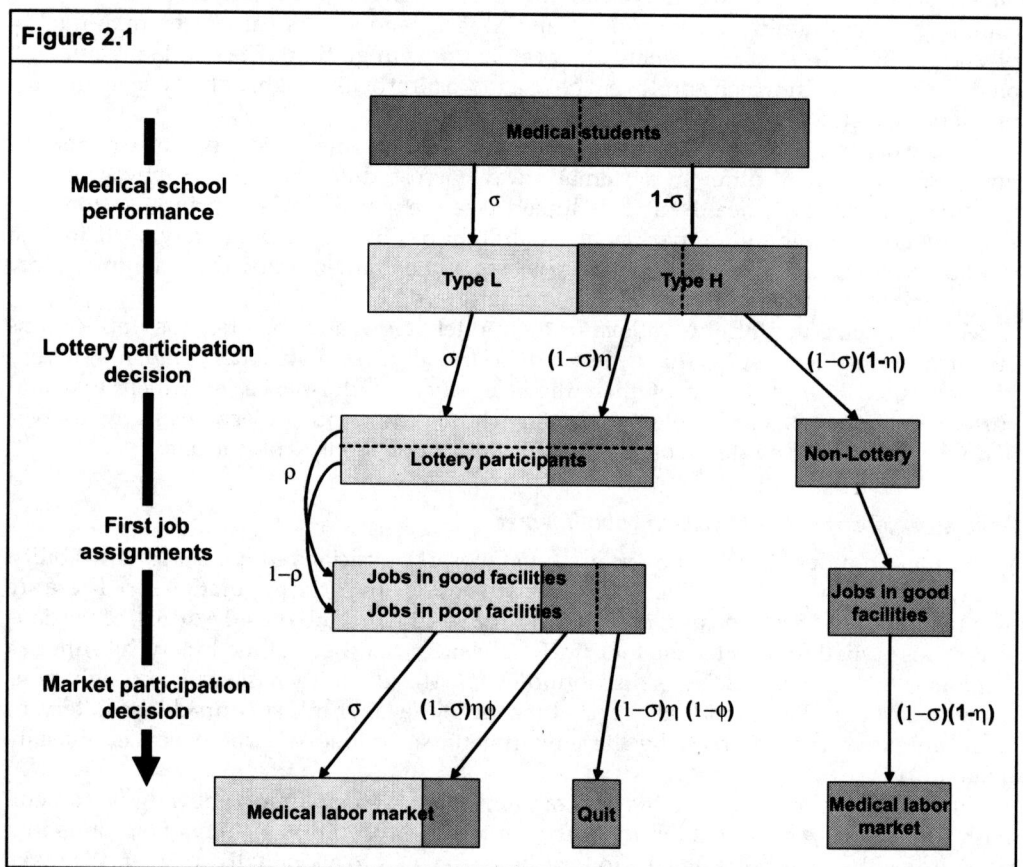

Figure 2.1

Without loss of generality, assume that all type L physicians have the same outside option, which is strictly less than their productivity in the profession, π_L. On the other hand, type H physicians have an outside option equal to $\tilde{\pi}_H + \mu$, where $\tilde{\pi}_H < \pi_H$ and μ is randomly distributed according to cdf F, with mean zero (so, on average, the outside option is less than a type H physician's productivity in the job), and finite support. Let us assume that $\max_\mu (\tilde{\pi}_H + \mu) < \pi_H$, so it is Pareto optimal for all type H physicians to continue in the profession.

A type H physician from the lottery will not enter the market for the second job and take his outside option instead as long as

$$\tilde{\pi}_H + \mu > \bar{\pi},$$

which occurs with probability $1 - F(\bar{\pi} - \tilde{\pi}_H) \equiv 1 - \phi(\bar{\pi})$. The number of H-type physicians from the lottery who enter in the market is then $(1 - \sigma)\eta\phi$. Since $\pi_H > \pi_L$, the average productivity of type L lottery participants who stay in the market is at least as high as the outside option they face, so the total number of lottery participants who stay in the market is

$$n_{in}^{Lott} = \underbrace{\sigma}_{L-\text{types}} + \underbrace{(1-\sigma)\eta\phi(\bar{\pi})}_{H-\text{types}}.$$

The average productivity of all physicians (both type L and type H) who were in the lottery and who enter the market is

$$\bar{\pi} = \frac{1}{n_{in}^{Lott}} \left[\sigma\pi_L + (1-\sigma)\eta\phi(\bar{\pi})\pi_H \right]. \tag{1}$$

This equation can be rearranged to yield

$$\bar{\pi} - \pi_L = \left(\frac{1-\sigma}{\sigma} \right) \eta\phi(\bar{\pi}) \left[\pi_H - \bar{\pi} \right]$$

At $\bar{\pi} = \pi_L$, the right-hand side of this expression is strictly positive, while the left-hand side is zero. At $\bar{\pi} = \pi_H$, the left-hand side is positive, and the right-hand side is zero. A sufficient condition for a unique solution to exist is that the right-hand side be strictly decreasing in $\bar{\pi}$ between π_L and π_H. This, in turn, can be guaranteed if

$$\frac{\phi'(\bar{\pi})}{\phi(\bar{\pi})} = \frac{f(\bar{\pi} - \tilde{\pi}_H)}{F(\bar{\pi} - \tilde{\pi}_H)} < \frac{1}{\pi_H - \bar{\pi}}$$

in this range. The right-hand side of this expression attains its smallest value (in the range $[\pi_L, \pi_H]$) at $\bar{\pi} = \pi_L$. So for given properties of the distribution function F, as long as π_H is not too much larger than π_L, there will be a unique solution to (1), which depends on π_L, π_H, and $\tilde{\pi}_H$ as well as σ and η.

Note that for a fixed value of η, as outside opportunities improve for type H physicians— i.e., as $\tilde{\pi}_H$ increases—the equilibrium value of $\bar{\pi}$ falls as a greater share of type H physicians from the lottery pool quit the market. In addition, however, the share of type H physicians who enter the lottery to begin with (for the first job) will fall. Taking π_L, π_H, $\tilde{\pi}_H$, and σ as parametric, η is the only endogenous variable, so let us write the equilibrium average productivity of lottery participants who enter the medical market after their first jobs as $\bar{\pi}(\eta)$.

To determine the share of type H physicians who initially enter the lottery, η, note that when type H physicians from the lottery are deciding whether to enter the market for their second job, they compare the wage $\bar{\pi}$ with their outside option $\tilde{\pi}_H + \mu$. If $\mu > \bar{\pi} - \tilde{\pi}_H$, then they do not enter the market and earn $\tilde{\pi}_H + \mu$; If $\mu < \bar{\pi} - \tilde{\pi}_H$, then they enter the market and earn $\bar{\pi}$. Thus the expected future wage for a type H physician who chooses to initially enter the lottery is

$$\bar{w}_H(\eta) = \frac{1}{n^{Lott}} \left(n_{in}^{Lott} \times \bar{\pi} + n_{out}^{Lott} \times \left[\tilde{\pi}_H + \int_{\bar{\pi} - \tilde{\pi}_H}^{\infty} \mu dF(\mu) \right] \right) \tag{2}$$

where $n_{out}^{Lott} = n^{Lott} - n_{in}^{Lott}$. Note that we assume that If μ is only revealed to a type H physician at the beginning for his second job search and is therefore not known when he decides whether to enter the lottery or not for his first job. The expected wage of a type H physician not in the lottery is simply π_H.

Because $\bar{\pi} \geq \pi_L$, all type L physicians enter the lottery. Type H physicians enter the lottery as long as

$$\bar{w}_H > \pi_H - \varepsilon,$$

where ε is the cost of not participating in the lottery. That is, H types participate in the lottery as long as $\varepsilon > \pi_H - \bar{w}_H$. Thus the share of type H physicians who enter the lottery is

$$\eta(\bar{w}_H) = 1 - G(\pi_H - \bar{w}_H). \tag{3}$$

Solving (2) and (3) gives the equilibrium share of type H physicians who participate in the lottery, η^*, and their expected future wage, $\bar{w}_H^*$, as illustrated in Figure 1.7.

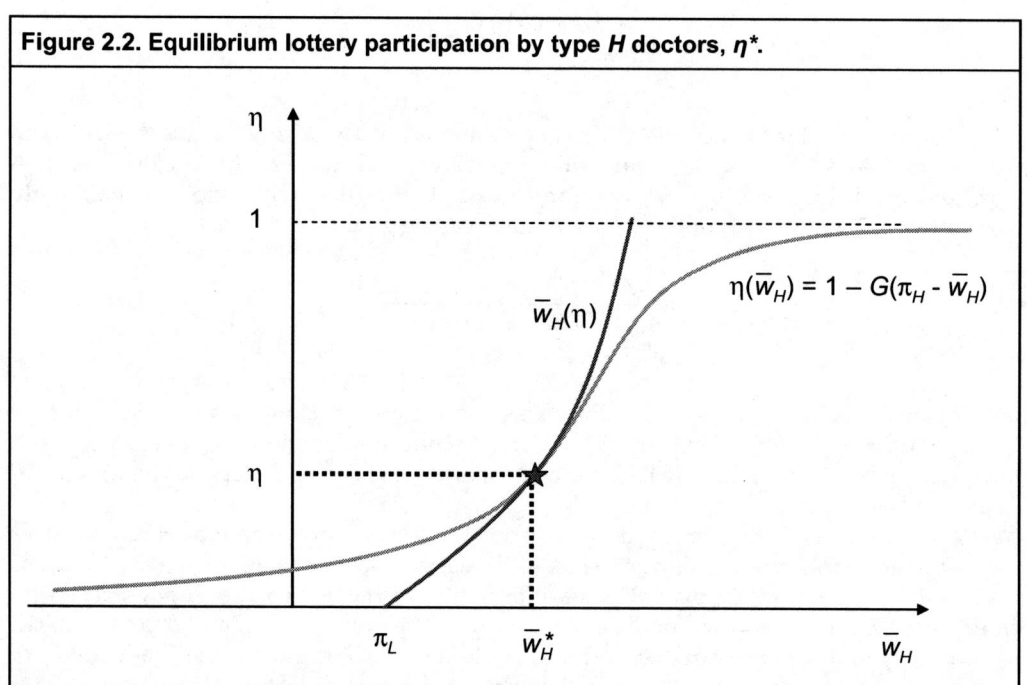

Figure 2.2. Equilibrium lottery participation by type *H* doctors, η^*.

Empirical Implications of the Model

The model above includes a number of empirically testable assumptions and predictions. The assumptions and some of the predictions relate to short-term effects, immediately following completion of physician training. Other predictions reflect the longer-term evolution of physicians' career paths.

- Main assumptions:

    1. There are regional differences in monetary and/or non-monetary returns that favor working in Addis.
    2. When the market allocates new graduates to jobs in different regions, this allocation is based at least in part on a worker's ability and locational preferences. Under the lottery, these variables do not predict the initial assignment across regions.

- Short-term predictions:

    1. High-ability physicians are more likely than low-ability physicians to opt out of the lottery.
    2. Growth of demand for private-sector services increase outside options and should therefore be associated with falling lottery participation.
    3. If the lottery assigns graduates randomly, then physicians assigned to Addis should have higher job satisfaction in their first assignment.

- Long-term predictions:

    1. Among high-ability physicians, current wages should be lower for lottery participants than for those who did not participate in the lottery.
    2. In light of this, rates of attrition among high-ability physicians should be higher for lottery participants than for those who did not participate in the lottery.

Empirical Setup: Sampling, Data, and Model Validity

In this section we review our sampling methodology, present descriptive statistics, and confirm the basic empirical assumptions of our model regarding the attractiveness of working in Addis Ababa and the workings of the job allocation mechanisms, both inside and outside the lottery system.

Sampling Methodology

Our sampling strategy aimed at obtaining representative samples of doctors from three of Ethiopia's eleven regions—the capital city of Addis Ababa, and two more remote regions of Tigray and the SNNPR. Addis is a city of about 3 million people and is located in the central highlands. Tigray has a population of about 4 million people and lies in the north of the country, bordering Eritrea, while the SNNPR, with a population of 14 million, lies to the southwest of Addis and borders Kenya to the south. The regional capital of Tigray is Mekele, and that of the SNNPR is Awassa. Our sample is representative within these geographic areas.[5] The design oversampled physicians in the SNNPR and Tigray due to the small number of physicians outside Addis Ababa: all physicians in these rural regions were sampled, while only about one third of physicians in Addis were. Our final sample included 219 physicians working in health centers and hospitals.

A random sample of one third of doctors was achieved in Addis Ababa by (a) randomly sampling facilities of the various types with sampling weights corresponding to the

Table 2.1. Numbers of Facilities and Physicians Surveyed

	Addis Ababa	SNNPR	Tigray	Total
Total sampled facilities with physicians	39	21	17	77
Hospitals	3	12	11	26
Health centers and clinics	36	9	6	51
Sampled physicians	91	72	56	219

estimated proportion of doctors working across the different facilities, and (b) interviewing all doctors at the sampled facilities. In the SNNPR and Tigray, all doctors were included in the sample. This was achieved by sampling all public hospitals in the SNNPR and Tigray (there are generally no doctors in non-hospital health facilities in these regions, and there were no private hospitals). In addition to interviewing health workers, we administered a facility-level survey with the facility administrator or other senior official at each facility we visited. A summary of our physician sample is provided in Table 1.3.

Among doctors, the interview response rate varied across regions: 86% in Tigray, while in the SNNPR and Addis Ababa it was lower—58% and 66%, respectively. However, exluding doctors on leave, the response rate was considerably higher. In Addis, the response rates were similar among public and private facilities (70% versus 64%, respectively), but the reasons differed. At public facilities, all doctors present agreed to be interviewed, although 21% of sampled doctors were absent on the day of the interview for unexplained reasons, and 9% for planned leave). In contrast to public facilities, the share of sampled doctors who were present but refused to be interviewed was 22% at private facilities. Further, no unexplained absences were recorded, while 15% of doctors were absent on planned leave. In Tigray, non-response arose because one sampled facility no longer existed, and one was inaccessible for security reasons. In the SNNPR, 9 out of 10 of the physicians listed as being employed but not interviewed were absent at the time of the facility visit for training purposes.

Description of Data

In this section we report summary statistics from both the facility and individual questionnaires, with a view to presenting a picture of working conditions and the physician labor force in the three regions covered by the survey. Table 1.4 provides summary statistics from the facility survey, weighted by the estimated share of physicians working in each type of facility. Doctors in the SNNPR and Tigray work in remote locations: they are 6 hours and 5.3 hours from their regional capitals respectively, which are themselves remote from Addis. However, the table shows that at least along several measurable inputs, facilities in the outlying regions are no worse than public facilities in Addis. In fact, SNNPR and Tigray facilities are better equipped to test for HIV and are more likely to have sufficient water supply. There are, in turn, differences between the two regions: for example, only half the doctors in Tigray work in facilities with sufficient medicine, compared with 88% of those in the SNNPR. Similarly, Tigray has more inpatient beds per doctor and more outpatients than both the SNNPR and public facilities in Addis.

Private facilities in Addis, on the other hand, are much smaller, with about half the number of inpatients and outpatients per doctor compared with public facilities in the capital. Some quality indicators, such as water availability, are reported as significantly better in Addis' private facilities, but on other dimensions private facilities report being either no better (equipment), or somewhat worse (medicine).

Demographic and economic data from the individual-level questionnaires are reported in Table 2.3. The top portion of that table shows that doctors in Addis Ababa, especially those working in the private sector, are more experienced than those in the regions. In

Table 2.2. Facility-Level Information, Based on Interviews with an Administrator, for Facilities with at Least One Physician

	All surveyed regions	Addis Ababa		SNNPR	Tigray
		Public	Private*		
Facility size					
Number of physicians (est.)	848	217	380	189	62
Physicians per facility	3.8	6.9	2.6	5.2	2.6
	(4.9)	(10.6)	(2.4)	(4.8)	(2.2)
Number inpatient beds	79.5	141.5	21.5	114.5	121.3
	(91.7)	(112.2)	(40.1)	(63.5)	(105.6)
Number inpatient beds per physician	20.9	20.5	8.3	22.0	46.7
Number outpatients	104.4	181.5	38.0	139.8	143.9
	(93.3)	(86.9)	(43.0)	(77.0)	(106.8)
Number outpatients per physician	27.5	26.3	14.6	26.9	55.3
Hours travel to regional capital	—	—	—	6.0	5.3
				(5.5)	(5.0)
Facility conditions (%)					
Reliable electricity/phone	99.3	100	100	97.4	97.9
Functioning X-ray machine	91.3	77.0	81.6	85.2	83.3
Functioning laboratory	100	100	100	100.0	100.0
Functioning operating theatre	62.1	61.8	42.6	92.6	97.9
Equipment to test for HIV	83.6	66.4	86.8	92.6	100
Sufficient water supply	74.5	23.0	96.0	87.3	85.4
Sufficient medicine	79.1	88.5	72.9	88.4	50.0
Sufficient equipment	87.1	83.9	84.5	100.0	70.8

* Includes for-profit and nonprofit NGO and missionary facilities.

Statistics are calculated using frequency weights corresponding to total number of doctors by region working in (1) public hospitals, (2) private hospitals, (3) government health centers, and (4) private, NGO, or missionary clinics.

Addis, men are somewhat over-represented in the private sector, while in the SNNPR there are virtually no female doctors whatsoever. We find evidence that doctors are more likely to have moved away from their home region to Addis than to either of the regions. This is reflected in the fact that three quarters of those in Tigray reported having lived there at age 10, compared with 53% in the SNNPR, and about 43% in Addis.

In economic terms, doctors in Addis do better than those in the regions. As reported in the bottom part of Table 2.3, asset ownership is higher in Addis, with one half and one quarter of the doctors working in private and public facilities, respectively, reporting ownership of a car, compared with less than 2% and 5%, respectively, in the SNNPR and Tigray. House ownership is higher among private-sector physicians in Addis (35%), but the rates among other doctors are similar (10–16%).

Table 2.4 reports labor market characteristics of sampled physicians. Salaries in Addis, especially among those working in the private sector, are considerably higher than those

Table 2.3. Demographic and Economic Characteristics of Sampled Health Workers

	All	Addis		SNNPR	Tigray
		Public	Private		
Demographics					
Share female (%)	17.1	30.0	16.0	2.6	26.8
Share married (%)	55.5	61.3	74.0	33.3	45.2
Age (years)	36.1	39.2	41.2	29.3	31.5
	(0.90)	(1.64)	(1.78)	(1.16)	(1.61)
Birth order	*	2.81	3.55	2.70	3.10
	*	(0.12)	(0.33)	(0.35)	(0.22)
Number of siblings	6.4	6.1	6.5	6.4	6.6
	(0.19)	(0.31)	(0.37)	(0.26)	(0.62)
Number of children	1.01	0.90	1.68	0.44	0.71
	(0.11)	(0.14)	(0.22)	(0.22)	(0.20)
Share with no children (%)	52.6	48.5	28.0	82.1	61.6
Number of children (for those with)	2.14	1.75	2.33	2.48	1.85
	(0.15)	(0.15)	(0.23)	(0.54)	(0.20)
Family connections to profession (%)					
Parents Health Workers	1.8	5.2	0.0	0.85	2.3
Siblings Health Workers	18.2	14.8	18.0	20.5	19.8
Other family Health Workers	18.5	19.9	26.0	13.7	7.0
Live in same region as at age 10	50.2	44.1	42.0	53.0	75.6
Assets (%)					
Own a car		26.9	51.0	1.9	4.8
Own land		14.8	4.1	13.9	2.4
Own house		15.2	34.7	10.2	15.7

earned in the SNNPR and Tigray. Doctors working in the public sector in Addis earn salaries about 50% more than the average doctor in the regions, while salaries of private-sector doctors are three times as much. The gap between private-sector salaries in Addis and those of other doctors is partly offset by additional sources of income: public-sector doctors in Addis earn additional income equal to 22% of their salaries, while the figures in the SNNPR and Tigray are 17% and 33% respectively, and between a third and a half of doctors in the regions outside Addis report receiving housing allowances (although we do not have data on the monetary value of these allowances). Indeed, significant shares of doctors working outside the Addis private sector report holding more than one job—from 23% in the Addis public sector, to 12% in Tigray. On the other hand, private-sector doctors in Addis supplement their (much higher) salaries by only 3%. Finally, physician household incomes are higher in Addis than elsewhere.

Part of the salary premium observed in Addis reflects higher rates of specialization among doctors there—about 40% compared with 20% in Tigray and just 7% in the SNNPR.

Table 2.4. Incomes and Assets of Sampled Health Workers

	All	Addis		SNNPR	Tigray
		Public	Private		
Incomes					
Salary (US$)	284.5	244.6	480.5	156.4	176.6
	(17.4)	(10.5)	(39.0)	(14.8)	(13.9)
Total income of health worker (US$)	320.9	297.0	496.8	181.4	233.1
	(24.8)	(24.8)	(40.1)	(29.7)	(38.2)
Total income of household (US$)	443.8	509.2	696.9	196.3	264.3
	(28.1)	(49.1)	(55.7)	30.0	(46.8)
Other compensation with job (%)	52.7	29.3	46.0	85.5	53.5
Housing allowance (%)	18.9	0.0	0.0	52.1	34.8
Type of job (%)					
Primary job in the private sector	36.9	0.0	100	9.4	0.0
Holds more than one job	**	23.5	20.4	16.7	12.0
Specialist	27.8	40.4	38.0	6.8	19.8
Institutional features (%)					
Participated in the lottery	57.4	62.0	56.0	54.7	58.1
Medical training sponsored by federal government	71.4	67.7	80.0	70.1	59.3
Applied for official release from public sector	44.9	38.7	86.0	19.7	4.7
of whom, release granted	84.1	73.9	95.3	47.8	25.0

However, we find that the rates of specialization in the public and private sectors in Addis are virtually identical, suggesting that training is not the sole driver of observed income differentials.

Finally, a similar proportion across the four employment categories, about 57%, reports having participated in the lottery, and between 59% and 80% of doctors had their medical training sponsored by the federal government (as opposed to a regional or foreign government, or a private sponsor). Lastly, the table shows the proportion of physicians who applied to receive an official release formally authorizing them to work in the private sector. Of those currently working in the private sector, most (86%) report having applied for this release, with the vast majority having been successful (95%). The corresponding application numbers are much lower among physicians working in the public sector—39%, 20%, and 5%, respectively, for Addis, the SNNPR, and Tigray, and their success rates are lower too—74%, 48%, and 25%, respectively.

Testing the Model's Assumptions

We begin by testing the main assumptions of the model regarding (i) the attractiveness of working in Addis relative to the regions, and (ii) the observable determinants of the location of physicians' first jobs, and how they differ between lottery participants and non-participants.

Job Satisfaction from Working in Addis

Pre-survey discussions with health workers suggest that the average physician perceives significant net benefits, in terms of salary and urban amenities, from working in Addis. This suggests that wages are not flexible enough to reduce these benefits to zero, or that physician jobs in Addis are qualitatively different than those in rural regions. The simple unconditional mean comparisons in Table 2.4, above, particularly with regard to wage differentials, support this notion. It is also consistent with separate work on the same sample of physicians by Hanson and Jack (2008), who find that relatively large financial incentives are necessary to induce sizeable shifts in physician labor to rural areas.

We confirm the attraction of working in the capital by estimating the relationship between having a job in Addis and wages, incomes, and job satisfaction, controlling for observable physician characteristics such as ability (as measured by academic class rank) and experience, and several other individual characteristics. We estimate an equation of the form

$$y_i = \beta_0 + \beta_1 D_i^{Addis} + x_i'\gamma + \varepsilon_i,$$

where x_i is a vector of characteristics of physician i, D_i^{Addis} is a dummy variable indicating whether physician i works in Addis, and y_i represents an employment characteristic such as wages, or a measure of job satisfaction. Conditional on x_i and assuming no omitted variable bias, the coefficient β_1 should be 0 or even negative if y_i is a measure of wages and the compensating wage differential framework holds. A positive value of β_1 indicates there are net benefits to having a job in Addis.

The results, reported in Table 2.5, confirm that differences in labor market outcomes between Addis and the regions remain, even conditional on a vector of observables. We find that physicians currently working in Addis earn salaries that are between 78% and 82% higher, and are considerably more content with various aspects of their work, especially those who are currently working in Addis and who initially participated in the lottery. Note that non-lottery physicians currently working in Addis are significantly more content with their jobs overall than their non-lottery counterparts working in the rural regions, despite *not* being more content about their much higher salaries, their workload, and their training opportunities. This suggests that Addis Ababa is also likely to have favorable non-employment characteristics. In sum, these tables support a main assumption of the model that on average, a job in Addis is more attractive than one outside the capital.

Determinants of First Job Assignments: Lottery versus Market

We next look at the determinants of first job assignment. If the lottery is random, we should find no significant predictors of first job assignment. On the other hand, if jobs in Addis are rationed, then market allocation might be correlated with certain individual characteristics. We limit the sample to doctors at least two years out of medical school. This is the sample used below when looking at longer-term outcomes. About 59% of physicians in our sample participated in the lottery, of whom about 11% were assigned to a first job in Addis Ababa. None of these swapped their assignment with other lottery participants. However, among the 89% of doctors assigned to one of the rural regions, 21% swapped their assignments with someone else, also assigned to one of the rural regions. In other words, there is some post-lottery sorting across rural regions. Among the others assigned to the rural region who did not swap, 2% still reported having their first job in Addis. We will use the assignment itself (intention to treat), not whether the actual first posting was in Addis, in the analyses below, unless otherwise noted. Among non-lottery physicians, 20% found their first job in Addis. We run separate regressions for the two sub-samples (lottery and non-lottery [market]), the results of which are reported in Table 2.6.[6]

The results confirm that the determinants of first job assignments differ systematically between lottery and non-lottery participants. Indeed, in line with the model, assignment appears to follow a market principle among non-lottery physicians, but not among

Table 2.5. Impact of currently working in Addis on physician job characteristics and satisfaction.

	Lottery	Market
Current salary (log)	0.821***	0.780***
	(0.144)	(0.167)
Current income (log)	0.733***	0.767***
	(0.176)	(0.157)
Doctor is specialized	0.289**	0.352***
	(0.112)	(0.131)
Satisfaction with current wage	0.943**	0.774
	(0.455)	(0.577)
Satisfaction with current training opportunities	-0.050	-0.480
	(0.310)	(0.422)
Satisfaction with current workload	0.773**	0.558
	(0.303)	(0.393)
Overall satisfaction with job	0.651*	0.809**
	(0.386)	(0.368)
Number of observations	120	85

Notes: Lottery includes those who participated in the lottery, whereas market includes those who did not. Each cell represents a separate OLS (Ordinary Least Squares) estimation (rows one and two) or (ordered) probit estimation (rows three to seven) and reports the coefficient on a dummy variable indicating whether the current job is in Addis (1) or one of the two regions (0). The dependent variable is in the left-hand column. Other controls are: class rank, family connections with the profession, sponsor, gender, experience, siblings, and birth order. Standard errors corrected for clustering at facility level.

*** Statistically significant at 1%-level

** Statistically significant at 5%-level

* Statistically significant at 10%-level

lottery physicians, under the assumption that employment in Addis is favorable. Among physicians who opted out of the lottery, those who report ranking in the second and third quintiles are respectively 21 and 25 percentage points less likely to find a first job in Addis Ababa, compared to those who ranked in the top quintile.[7] Social connection to the medical profession, as proxied by having a relative working in the sector, also improves a non-lottery participant's chance of securing employment in Addis. In sum, it is both *what* and *who* you know that helps secure a job in the capital.[8]

On the other hand, as expected, class rank is not a significant determinant of job assignment among lottery participants, and neither does connection to the profession influence the chance of such individuals being posted to Addis or the regions. Nevertheless, the second and third columns of the table do show that assignment within the lottery is not entirely random: physicians whose medical studies were sponsored by regional authorities are 12.5% less likely to have a first job assignment in Addis than lottery physicians whose studies were sponsored by the federal government. We interpret this as reflecting the discretion of officials in charge of the national lottery to give regions priority in recruiting those graduates whose medical training they funded. The only other variable correlated with the job assignment of lottery participants is sex: men are 26.2 percentage points less likely to be assigned to Addis than women. This difference could reflect preferences on both the demand and supply sides: first, Hanson and Jack (2008) find that the value of a job in Addis Ababa is significantly higher for women than for men; and second (and perhaps

Table 2.6. Predicting Assignment to Addis Ababa in First Job after Medical School

	Predicting first job in Addis Ababa				
	Lottery		Market		
	I	II	III	IV	V
Second-ranked student	0.094	0.063		-0.176126	-0.210126
	(0.079)	(0.070)		(0.117)	(0.134)
Third-ranked student	0.038	0.045		-0.304*	-0.250**
	(0.102)	(0.103)		(0.151)	(0.124)
Parents health workers	-0.007	-0.001		-0.348*	-0.261**
	(0.087)	(0.082)		(0.195)	(0.120)
Other relatives health workers	0.055	0.082		0.265**	0.303***
	(0.107)	(0.107)		(0.129)	(0.106)
Sponsor: regional authorities	-0.180***	-0.161**	-0.125**	0.024	
	(0.064)	(0.065)	(0.058)	(0.100)	
Sponsor: private/foreign government	0.136	0.103	0.087	0.017	
	(0.111)	(0.096)	(0.088)	(0.165)	
Male (=1)	-0.250***	-0.256***	-0.262***	-0.126	
	(0.086)	(0.087)	(0.083)	(0.175)	
Years experience	0.004	0.001		-0.007	
	(0.018)	(0.016)		(0.019)	
Years experience squared	-0.000	-0.000		0.000	
	(0.001)	(0.001)		(0.001)	
Order of birth	0.001	0.006		0.035	
	(0.015)	(0.014)		(0.029)	
Number of siblings	0.010	0.009		-0.024	
	(0.017)	(0.017)		(0.032)	
Observations	122	122	122	85	85
R-squared	0.1577	0.1764	0.1341	0.2244	0.1916

Linear probability model. In columns I, IV, and V the dependent variable is the actual location of the first job (Addis=1), whereas in columns II and III it is the location of the first job as assigned under the lottery.

Standard errors corrected for clustering at facility level. -values: *** 1%, ** 5%, * 10%, ~15%.

related) we do not rule out the possibility that the regional authorities in Addis submit physician openings specifically targeting female graduates.

In the following two sections, we turn to empirical tests of both the short-run and long-run implications of the model.

Short-Run Impacts of the Lottery System on the Physician Labor Market

Who Participates in the Lottery?

While lottery participation has officially been mandatory, as we observed above, many physicians in our sample did not get their first job through this mechanism. The model predicts that high-ability physicians should be more likely to select out of the lottery than low-ability physicians. This is tested in the first column of Table 2.7. Indeed, third-ranked

Table 2.7. Determinants of Lottery Participation, Private Sector Work, and Specialization

	Lottery participation			Currently in private sector		Physician is specialized	Salary (log)
	I	II	III	IV	V	VI	VII
Second-ranked student	0.031	0.032	-0.071	-0.175*		-0.233***	-0.174
	(0.093)	(0.092)	(0.098)	(0.093)		(0.082)	(0.112)
Third-ranked student	0.245***	0.245***	0.242***	-0.179126		-0.303***	-0.137
	(0.092)	(0.092)	(0.091)	(0.112)		(0.080)	(0.125)
Parents health workers	-0.032	-0.021	0.110	-0.235*	-0.195**	-0.204***	-0.236
	(0.231)	(0.230)	(0.145)	(0.129)	(0.093)	(0.075)	(0.181)
Other relatives	-0.049	-0.046	-0.122	0.122	0.131	-0.184***	0.189
health workers	(0.108)	(0.107)	0.107	(0.096)	(0.102)	(0.057)	(0.117)
Sponsor:	-0.246*	-0.250*	-0.220	-0.206**	-0.207**	-0.212***	-0.148
regional authorities	(0.134)	(0.133)	(0.140)	(0.099)	(0.099)	(0.051)	(0.104)
Sponsor:	-0.417***	-0.415***	-0.448***	-0.220**	-0.241**	0.162	-0.206**
private/foreign govt	(0.111)	(0.112)	(0.110)	(0.105)	(0.108)	(0.162)	(0.099)
Male (=1)	0.014	0.012	-0.004	0.104	0.092	0.126*	-0.027
	(0.118)	(0.118)	(0.121)	(0.093)	(0.093)	(0.073)	(0.097)
Years experience	0.061***	0.060***	0.070***	0.027	0.028	0.000	0.051***
	(0.015)	(0.015)	(0.014)	(0.018)	(0.018)	(0.004)	(0.016)
Years experience^2	-0.002***	-0.002***	-0.002***	-0.000	-0.000		-0.001***
	(0.000)	(0.000)	(0.000)	(0.001)	(0.000)		(0.000)
Order of birth	-0.068***	-0.066***	-0.061**	0.029	0.018	0.073***	0.029
	(0.025)	(0.025)	(0.027)	(0.021)	(0.020)	(0.020)	(0.021)
Number of siblings	0.042**	0.041**	0.036*	-0.005	0.005	-0.059***	0.007
	(0.019)	(0.019)	(0.019)	(0.017)	(0.015)	(0.021)	(0.015)
Private clinics		-0.046	-0.519***				
common		(0.150)	(0.146)				
Second rank x Private			0.462***				
clinics common			(0.052)				
Third rank x Private			0.204				
clinics common			(0.305)				
Specialist training					0.123		0.695***
					(0.114)		(0.120)
Participated in lottery						-0.519***	
						(0.189)	
Lottery participant						0.136*	
x rank (linear)						(0.087)	
Observations	216	216	216	207	207	207	203
(Pseudo) R-squared	0.1581	0.1586	0.2110	0.2023	0.1840	0.2750	0.2690

Notes: Probit models (dprobit coefficients reported) for lottery participation, based on entire sample. Linear probability for private-sector participation (probit omits five observations whose parents were health workers because none of them work in the private sector). OLS for log salary. Private sector and specialization limited to physicians at least two years out of medical school.

*** Statistically significant at 1%-level

** Statistically significant at 5%-level

* Statistically significant at 10%-level

students are nearly 25 percentage points more likely to participate in the lottery than second- and first-ranked students.

The lottery is operated by the federal government, which also sponsored the training of 71% of the physicians in our sample. We find that these physicians are more likely to participate in the lottery, perhaps because they face a higher cost of opting out, given the federal government's sponsorship role. Specifically, physicians whose medical training was sponsored by regional authorities (who make up 12% of all physicians) were 25 percentage points less likely, and those sponsored privately or by foreign governments (who, combined, make up 16% of all physicians) were 42 percentage points less likely, to participate in the lottery than federally sponsored physicians.

Other determinants of lottery participation include family size (those from large families are more likely to participate) and birth order (those born later are less likely to participate), which may reflect differential costs (ε) of opting out of the lottery. The coefficients on years of experience (the number of years since graduation) reflect the general decline in lottery participation.

Impact of Private-Sector Growth on Lottery Participation

The growth of demand for private-sector services can similarly be interpreted as a reduction in the search or other utility costs, ε, associated with opting out of the lottery, and should therefore lead to a reduction in lottery participation. We take the demand for physician labor by the private sector as exogenous to any graduate's lottery participation decision. Columns II and III in Table 2.7 report our findings.

Although we lack comprehensive data on the rise of the private sector, surveyed physicians were asked whether private clinics were already fairly common at the time they started their medical training. We use their responses as a proxy for the size, and growth, of the private sector. Column II in Table 2.7 above shows that the coefficient estimate on this variable is not significantly different from zero. However, after introducing the interaction with class rank (column III), both the coefficient on the variable itself, and on its interaction with second rank, becomes very significant and large in size. In particular it suggests that, consistent with the model above, before the expansion of the private sector, lottery participation was no different between first- and second-ranked students, but 25 percentage points higher among third-ranked students—possibly because the lottery was perceived to increase the chances that a third-ranked doctor would get a job in Addis. After the expansion of the private sector, third-ranked students are still 25 percentage points more likely to participate than first-rank students, although both groups experience a large drop in participation of 52 percentage points. Second-ranked students, on the other hand, do not experience a decrease in lottery participation, which seems puzzling.

We can speculate on the forces behind this pattern of effects. One possibility is that physicians in general aim to enter the private sector at some point in their careers. First-ranked physicians expect to command a high salary immediately in the private sector, so they are willing to incur the costs of quitting the lottery. The estimation reported in column IV of Table 2.7 shows what factors determine whether a physician currently has his primary job in the private sector. Indeed, the private sector attracts the highest-ability physicians, as measured by their medical school ranking and their years of experience. Physicians in both the second and third quintile are about 18 percentage points less likely than physicians in the first quintile to work in the private sector.

However, as shown in the next column, it is not the case that doctors who undergo further training and specialize are more likely to be working in the private sector (both are choice variables, so this is merely presented as a correlation conditional on other variables). Still, as reported in the last column, column VII, physicians who specialize earn considerably higher wages (70% higher), even controlling for experience, rank, and other background variables. Column VI seeks to reconcile these facts. In particular, it shows that while lower-ranked physicians and physicians participating in the lottery are less likely to specialize, the gap in specialization rates between lottery and non-lottery physicians declines with class rank. For second- and third-ranked physicians, the probability of receiving specialization training is very similar inside and outside the lottery, and similar to those of first-ranked physicians inside the lottery. The fact that there is no significant difference across the ranks within the lottery is consistent with our model of adverse selection.[9]

In sum, the rise of the private sector provides a clear incentive for first-ranked physicians to leave the lottery; doing so not only allows them to take advantage of private-sector opportunities, but significantly increases their chance of receiving specialization training, thus raising their public-sector wage opportunities. By the same reasoning, the growth of the private sector should also strengthen the incentives of second- and third-ranked physicians to quit the lottery—although to a lesser degree, since leaving the lottery is not associated with improved specialization training prospects. The reason private-sector growth has *not* increased lottery exit among second-rank physicians remains unclear.

Initial Job Satisfaction of Lottery Participants and Non-Participants

Within the group of lottery participants, we expect satisfaction with the first assignment to be higher among those who were (randomly) assigned to high-valued jobs such as those in Addis, compared with those who were (randomly) assigned to the rural regions. This is explored in Table 2.8, which provides OLS, ordered probit, and nearest neighbor matching (NNM) estimates of the short-term sample average treatment effects (Abadie and Imbens, 2002) of having a first job *assignment* to Addis Ababa, controlling for background variables such as class rank, sponsor, etc. We estimate the impact of initial job assignment for the two sub-samples (lottery and non-lottery participants), assuming that any selection into Addis is on observables. This identifying assumption is clearly

Table 2.8. The Short-Term Impact of Having a First Job in Addis Ababa

	Lottery		Market	
	OLS/OProbit I	NNM II	OLS/OProbit III	NNM IV
Duration (years) first job	1.092***	2.625***	1.957**	3.275***
	(0.364)	(0.338)	(0.798)	(0.970)
Wage satisfaction, first job	-0.048	-0.362*	0.558	-2.012***
	(0.467)	(0.195)	(0.500)	(0.382)
Training satisfaction, first job	-0.375	-3.535***	0.004	0.871***
	(0.507)	(0.142)	(0.609)	(0.209)
Work load satisfaction, first job	0.204	-0.376**	0.086	-0.339
	(0.286)	(0.161)	(0.301)	(0.313)
Overall satisfaction, first job	0.483	3.518***	0.154	-1.766***
	(0.394)	(0.382)	(0.576)	(0.399)
Number of observations	121	121	85	85

Notes: Each cell represents a separate OLS (duration), ordered probit (satisfaction), or NNM with robust std errors and bias correction estimation and reports the coefficient on a dummy variable equal to one if the first job assignment was in Addis. Dependent variables are in the first column. Controls are dummies for class rank, parents or relatives who are health workers, medical school sponsor, gender, experience, experience^2, number of siblings, and birth order. All estimations exclude physicians less than two years out of medical school.

p-values: *** 1%, ** 5%, * 10%, ~15%. Ordered probit std errors corrected for clustering at facility level.

tenuous among non-lottery participants, since there could be unobserved covariates that are correlated with the initial Addis assignment but independent of an individual's class rank and whether he or she has relatives in the health profession. Our main focus is therefore on the lottery sample.[10]

The main result is shown in the bottom row: among physicians who participated in the lottery (columns I and II), the ordered probit and NNM estimates are both positive, indicating higher overall first-job satisfaction for those initially assigned to Addis, although only the latter is significant. Similarly, none of the other ordered probits for the satisfaction variables are significant, while the NNM estimates indicate that lottery participants assigned to Addis were significantly *less* satisfied with their wages, training opportunities, and workload. As mentioned above, this result has an interesting parallel with the findings by Cullen et al. (2006), who find that prospective high school students winning a lottery that gave them the option of attending a high-performing school in Chicago did not seem to benefit, suggesting a potential mismatch not foreseen by lottery participants. That overall satisfaction was nevertheless significantly higher may be more of a reflection of non-work amenities provided by working in Addis than of the job itself. The results among market physicians (columns III and IV) are ambiguous. The ordered probit satisfaction estimates are similarly not significant, while the NNM suggests lower wage and overall satisfaction, but higher training satisfaction, for those who start their careers in the capital. Lastly, both ordered probit and NNM estimates indicate that the duration of the first assignment is significantly longer in Addis for lottery as well as market physicians.

Longer-Term Dynamics in the Physician Labor Market

We now turn to an examination of the longer-term impacts of initial job assignments early in the careers of physicians. The two aspects of first-job assignment we distinguish between are, first, *where* a physician is assigned and, second, *by which mechanism* he or she is assigned—i.e., lottery or market. That is, we first estimate the impact of getting a first job in Addis Ababa on future labor market outcomes, which will help shed light on the long-term private costs of assigning graduates to rural facilities. We then turn to the impact of the lottery itself on the workings of the labor market.

Long-Term Impact of Initial Assignment to Addis

Although jobs in Addis are more attractive because of the income and amenity values they provide, is getting such a posting early in one's career an important determinant of future labor market outcomes? In this sub-section we explore this issue, first using the lottery system as a quasi-randomized experiment to examine the impact on lottery participants, and then employing matching techniques to measure the impact on all physicians in our sample. Table 2.9 examines how the impact of having had a first job in Addis differs between lottery participants and non-participants.

The long-term impact is similar to the short-term one. Overall satisfaction is significantly higher for both the ordered probit and NNM estimate, despite signficantly lower chances of being specialized than doctors initally assigned by the lottery to one of the rural regions. In contrast, as shown in columns III and IV, both the OLS/ordered probit and NNM estimates indicate that market physicians with a first assignment in Addis are more likely to be specialized. One explanation for this difference is that Addis attracts high-ranking medical students through the market, with whom average-ranked lottery students must compete for specialist training. Perhaps related, lottery doctors assigned initially to Addis are not more likely to be currently employed there or have employment in the private sector.

The table shows further that, except for the specialization estimate, for market physicians the effects of getting a first job in Addis are unclear, as shown in columns III and IV. None of

Table 2.9. The Long-Term Impacts of Having a First Job in Addis Ababa

	Lottery		Market	
	OLS/OProbit I	NNM II	OLS/OProbit III	NNM IV
Current job in Addis	0.121	-0.025	0.036	0.388***
	(0.241)	(0.214)	(0.130)	(0.097)
Specialized	-0.158**	-0.165***	0.190*	0.412***
	(0.073)	(0.039)	(0.098)	(0.145)
Current job in private sector	0.195	0.266126	0.140	-0.620***
	(0.193)	(0.168)	(0.199)	(0.130)
Current salary (log)	0.140	0.465***	0.054	0.335**
	(0.199)	(0.173)	(0.184)	(0.155)
Overall satisfaction, current job	0.867*	1.720**	0.014	-3.058***
	(0.520)	(0.676)	(0.559)	(0.471)
Currently lives in same region	0.358***	0.271***	-0.130	-0.262***
as at age 10	(0.117)	(0.055)	(0.187)	(0.073)
Number of observations	121	121	85	85

Notes: Each cell represents a separate OLS, ordered probit (for satisfaction), or NNM with robust standard errors and bias correction estimation (Abadie and Imbens, 2002) and reports the coefficient on a dummy variable equal to one if the first job assignment was in Addis. Dependent variables are in the first column. Controls are dummies for class rank, parents or relatives who are health workers, medical school sponsor, gender, experience, experience[2], number of siblings, and birth order. All estimations exclude physicians less than two years out of medical school.

p-values: *** 1%, ** 5%, * 10%. Ordered probit std errors corrected for clustering at facility level.

the other coefficients on being first assigned to Addis in the OLS estimates are significant, while all NNM estimates are very significant yet unclear. They suggest that physicians landing a job in Addis after medical school are significantly more likely to still be working there, and earn higher incomes, but are less likely to work in the private sector and less satisfied with their current job. We are reluctant to interpret these non-lottery findings, not only because of likely omitted variable bias, but because these NNM non-lottery findings are very sensitive to the matching variables used.[11]

In sum, the estimates for those who participated in the lottery suggest that in the long run there is a fair amount of mobility following the initial assignment. Still, physicians assigned to Addis through the lottery may fare slightly better than those assigned to the rural area, as measured by their current job satisfaction. This is despite having lower levels of specialization than lottery physicians initially assigned to the rural regions. The bottom row in the table may be able to reconcile these findings. Physicians assigned to Addis are significantly more likely to be living now in the region in which they lived as adolescents, suggesting that despite lower specialization, they may benefit from non-employment-related compensating differences.

Evidence of Adverse Selection

Consistent with the notion that the lottery obscures important information, we found that differences in specialization rates between lottery participants and nonparticipants were smaller among low-ranked physicians than they were among high-ranked physicians. Next we investigate the extent to which the data further support the idea that the labor market in which lottery participants operate later in their careers suffers from adverse selection. We examine wage compression and labor market attrition.

Wages

If information on worker quality is publicly observable, then a physician's first job does not provide a useful signal to future employers. In our empirical analysis we allow for the possibility that working in Addis Ababa (either in a good facility or in a place with access to other colleagues and a richer learning environment) has a real, positive effect on productivity. In this case, conditioning on class rank, future wages may be positively correlated with having a first job in Addis. However, the distribution of wages should be the same for both lottery participants and those who enter the market immediately after graduation. On the other hand, if the lottery obfuscates worker-quality information, then we expect that the conditional wage distribution will be narrowed. Figure 1.7, which shows the unconditional wage distribution by rank separately for lottery and non-lottery physicians, provides suggestive evidence to this effect.

Consistent with the model, the graph shows that physicians who were third-ranked students earn virtually the same amount of money whether they were initially in the lottery or not. Among second-ranked, non-lottery physicians earn slightly more, but not much. However, there is a large difference among first-ranked physicians, with non-lottery physicians earning 39% more on average. Table 2.10 explores this in a regression context predicting log wages using interactions between class rank and lottery participation. Here, the third-rank category is omitted to focus on first-rank dynamics.

The table first shows that there is not enough power to include a dummy for lottery participation and its interaction with dummies for rank one and rank two—none of these are significant (column I). Forcing the effect of lottery participation to be zero for third-ranked physicians (consistent with Figure 1.7), the coefficient estimates on the interaction terms both fall just outside the significance range (column II). Combining first and second rank in their interaction with lottery participation, column III shows that compared with third-ranked physicians, second-ranked physicians earn 18% more if they are outside the lottery (p-value is 0.159), but earn the same as third-ranked physicians inside the lottery. On the other hand, first-ranked physicians earn 48% more than third-ranked physicians outside the lottery, but only 24% more inside the lottery (a combination of the direct and interaction effect). This is consistent with the model's prediction that there is substantial wage pooling within the lottery. It is conceivable that an omitted variable could bias our results, for instance if it acted both to increase wages and to induce individuals to opt out of the lottery. However we believe this is unlikely for two reasons. First, if this were the case, then one would expect third-ranked physicians to also earn more outside the lottery. And second, if there is no wage pooling inside the lottery, one would expect second-ranked students inside the lottery to earn more than third-ranked students inside the lottery.

Labor Market Attrition

Recall that among the pool of high-ability lottery physicians, those with high later-life reservation wages are predicted by the model to leave the profession, leading to adverse selection. Naturally, by the mere fact that we cannot observe physicians who left the population of physicians, finding evidence of attrition is challenging. Figure 1.8 and Table 2.11 provide two pieces of evidence that are, at a minimum, consistent.

First, the time series of lottery participation show a drop not just among the latest 2006 cohort, which is consistent with anecdotal evidence that the lottery is unraveling (we are unable to identify whether this change reflects a real drop in lottery participation, delayed attrition from the health sector by nonparticipants, or a combination of both), but also among the oldest cohorts before 1993. Because anecdotal evidence suggests that government enforcement of the lottery was greater in the past, one would expect that lottery

Table 2.10. Wage Evidence of Adverse Selection among Lottery Participants

	Log current salary		
	I	II	III
First-ranked student	0.421**	0.505***	0.476***
	(0.178)	(0.155)	(0.137)
Second-ranked student	0.067	0.153	0.178126
	(0.156)	(0.130)	(0.125)
First-ranked x lottery	-0.182	-0.291	
	(0.214)	(0.193)	
Second-ranked x lottery	-0.082	-0.196	
	(0.207)	(0.139)	
First and Second ranked			-0.240*
x lottery			(0.121)
Lottery	-0.116		
	(0.169)		
Parents healthworkers	-0.332	-0.344	-0.324
	(0.293)	(0.286)	(0.258)
Other relatives	0.061	0.064	0.067
health workers	(0.130)	(0.129)	(0.127)
Years experience	0.061***	0.058***	0.058***
	(0.020)	(0.019)	(0.019)
Years experience^2	-0.002***	-0.001***	-0.001***
	(0.001)	(0.001)	(0.001)
Sponsor:	-0.310*	-0.304*	-0.311*
regional authority	(0.165)	(0.164)	(0.163)
Sponsor:	-0.167	-0.158	-0.156
private/foreign govt.	(0.115)	(0.115)	(0.116)
Order of birth	0.066**	0.068**	0.070**
	(0.028)	(0.028)	(0.027)
Number of siblings	-0.020	-0.020	-0.022
	(0.019)	(0.018)	(0.019)
Observations	203	203	203
R-squared	0.2823	0.2810	0.2799

Notes: All estimations exclude physicians who were less than two years out of medical school. OLS estimations with standard errors corrected for clustering at facility level.

p-values: *** 1%, ** 5%, * 10%, ~15%, ~ = 0.159.

participation was highest among the oldest cohorts. If this was the case, then differential attrition rates between lottery and non-lottery participants over time could have given rise to this pattern.

Second, Table 2.11 below explores in a regression context the extent to which high-ranked lottery participants have left the profession more frequently than similar individuals who did not participate in the lottery.

Table 2.11. Attrition Evidence of Adverse Selection among Lottery Participants

	First-ranked
Lottery participation	0.142
	(0.139)
Lottery participation x experience	-0.020*
	(0.011)
Experience	0.035*
	(0.019)
Experience^2	-0.079126
	(0.050)
Number of observations	209

Notes: Robust standard errors clustered at the facility level. OLS estimation excludes physicians who were less than two years out of medical school.
p-values: * 10%, ~15%.

The dependent variable is a dummy for being first ranked. The positive coefficient on experience (0.035) indicates that older cohorts are more likely to be first ranked than younger cohorts, suggesting that over time first-ranked individuals have chosen not to enter the profession (in Ethiopia).[12] On the other hand, the negative coefficient on the interaction between experience and lottery participation indicates that within older cohorts, lottery participants in our sample are less likely to be first ranked than nonparticipants. This suggests that among high-ranked individuals, lottery participants have left the profession more frequently than nonparticipants. This is consistent with the idea that the lottery has long-term impacts on the workings of the physician labor market.

Conclusion

Delivering health and other public services to remote areas of developing countries is perhaps one of the greatest challenges facing poor countries that aspire to reach the Millennium Development Goals. This paper has used a newly collected dataset on Ethiopian physicians to shed light on issues of rural physician labor supply, including the dynamics of career evolution and the allocative efficiency of the physician labor market. We have used a lottery mechanism employed to assign medical school graduates to their first jobs to identify the long-term impact of initial postings to rural areas, and we have examined the performance of the physician labor market born of that lottery mechanism.

We find the market for new physicians operates surprisingly efficiently. Although new graduates are allocated randomly by the lottery, better graduates opt out of the lottery, especially since the rise of private health sector opportunities, and earn more in the short and long run than lower-quality physicians. And although the lottery is *ex ante* fair, *ex post* we find that physicians assigned through the lottery to Addis were more satisfied with their first assignment and remain more satisfied with their current assignment. However, we find that being posted under the lottery to a rural area is not the end of a physician's chances for a successful career; indeed, they are more successful in getting specialized training than lottery participants initially assigned to Addis, and they are no less likely to be currently working in Addis. In fact, there is some indication that doctors initially assigned to Addis through the lottery compete unsuccessfully with higher-ranked non-lottery doctors for specialization training and opt to move to their home regions instead. This suggests that the long-term costs of rural assignment are not especially high.

There is evidence that the lottery mechanism obfuscates information about worker quality, which can lead to adverse selection in the physician labor market later on. We find that among lottery participants, rates of specialization and wages are compressed. A high-ability physician participating in the lottery earns less and is less likely to be specialized compared with a similar physician who did not take part in the lottery. Consequently, there is some indirect evidence that better-ranked lottery participants are more likely to leave the profession over time. These observations support our hypothesis that the lottery has some negative long-run effects on the workings of the labor market, and could possibly contribute the medical brain drain. Enforcing full participation in the lottery is unlikely to ameliorate these effects. Instead, policy should focus on explicit financial or in-kind incentives to attract physicians to rural positions and to motivate them once there.

Notes

[1] Four, if we count the decision to enter medical school.

[2] The terminology suggests that rural work is akin to a prison sentence. The maximum number of health workers assigned to each region is decided before October by a three-person committee at the Ministry of Health, on the basis of the official requests of health workers sent by each region. An exception in the lottery system has recently been introduced with respect to the assignment to posts in the newest regions of Benishangul, Hafar, Somali, and Gambella. Before the lottery takes place, each health worker is asked whether he or she would be willing to work in any of these new regions. If the answer is negative, as in the majority of cases, the corresponding posts are added to the lottery.

[3] It would seem fairer to require all health workers to spend a given amount of time in undesirable jobs, rather than to randomly assign such tasks to an unlucky share.

[4] We show below that federally funded doctors are more likely to enter the lottery than those with private funding, suggesting that the threat of government sanctions is operative.

[5] Other regions, such as Oromia (which surrounds Addis Ababa) and Amhara (which is immediately north of Oromia), are larger (with 26 and 19 million residents, respectively) and less remote, at least in terms of direct distance measures, but we have no reason to expect this to have introduced systematic biases in our estimates.

[6] Linear probability estimation is used instead of probit maximum likelihood, since there are a few instances where probit estimations are forced to drop several observations. For example, in the lottery sample, there are three healthworkers whose parents were also healthworkers. Because all three work outside Addis, these are dropped in probit estimations.

[7] 39% of physicians report being in the first quintile, 41% in the second, and 20% in the third, with 0% in the fourth and fifth quintiles

[8] Somewhat surprisingly, doctors with a parent in the sector are *less* likely to get a first job in Addis. One reason might be that such doctors might be inclined to join their parentsí practices, which could be outside Addis.

[9] Specialization rates relative to first-ranked physicians outside the lottery: (1) first-ranked physician inside lottery (–37%); (2) second-ranked physician outside lottery (–23%) and inside lottery (–0.47%); and (3) third-ranked physician outside lottery (–29%) and inside lottery (–40%).

[10] Note that the small sample size (121 lottery observations) means that we are unlikely to detect relatively small differences in outcomes.

[11] For example, including only rank and whether parents and relatives have been health workers (the only correlates with initial Addis assignment) as matching variables, all estimates are insignificant (smallest p-value = 0.29), except specialization, which remains significantly positive

[12] Alternatively, it could be that younger cohorts of physicians are more humble in reporting their class rank. Because all the estimations control for experience, this would not affect our findings. Still, there is little reason to think that the younger generation is somehow more humble.

References

Cullen, J.B., B.A. Jacob, and S. Levitt. 2006. "The Effect of School Choice on Participants: Evidence from Randomized Lotteries." *Econometrica* 74 (5): 1191–1230.

Hanson, Kara and William Jack. 2008. "Health Worker Preferences for Job Attributes in Ethiopia: Results from a Discrete Choice Experiment," mimeo.

Kaufman, J. E., and J. E. Rosenbaum. 1992. "The Education and Employment of Low-Income Black Youth in White Suburbs." *Educational Evaluation and Policy Analysis* 14: 229–240. [1194,1224]

Light, A., and W. Strayer. 2000. "Determinants of College Completion: School Quality or Student Ability." *Journal of Human Resources* 35: 299–332. [1194,1224]

Ministry of Health, Government of Ethiopia. 2005. *Health and Health-Related Indicators: 1997.*

Niederle, M., and A. E. Roth. 2007. "The Effects of a Centralized Clearinghouse on Job Placement, Wages, and Hiring Practices." *NBER Working Paper* 13529.

Roth, A. E. 2007. "What Have We Learned from Market Design." *NBER Working Paper* 13530.

CHAPTER 3

Designing Incentives for Rural Health Workers

Kara Hanson and William Jack

Introduction

The supply and geographic distribution of health workers are major constraints to improving health in low-income countries. A number of recent studies have highlighted the shortage of skilled health workers in many settings (WHO 2006), the impact this has on health outcomes (Anand and Barnighausen 2004), and the risk this poses for the achievement of the Millenium Development Goals (WHO 2006; Joint Learning Initiative 2004). However, there remains limited evidence about what sorts of policies will attract nurses and doctors into medical training, improve the retention of trained health workers, and encourage them to work in rural areas where problems of inaccessibility of services are most acute.

A number of strategies have been employed to address the human resources challenge in low- and middle-income settings including compulsory rural service for new graduates (e.g. in South Africa); payment of incentives or "hardship allowances" for those posted to rural areas (as proposed in Rwanda); or encouraging self-selection by those with a commitment to rural service (as practiced, for example, in Thailand, Wilbulpolprasert and Pengpaibon 2003). Yet few of these strategies have been systematically evaluated, and the effectiveness of each will likely reflect country-specific labour market conditions, political systems, and culture and tradition.

The challenges of human development are particularly extreme in Ethiopia, a country with a population of over 70 million people, 85% of whom live in rural areas. It is one of the poorest countries in the world, with per capita income of about $150, and although the poverty rate has fallen by 8 percentage points over the last 10 years, it nonetheless remained at 37% in 2006. The country faces acute challenges in reaching all of the Millenium Development Goals, including the three goals relating to health—to reduce child mortality, improve maternal health, and combat HIV/AIDS, malaria, and other diseases. In 2005 the infant mortality rate was 77 per 1,000, the under-5 mortality rate was 123 per 1,000, and the maternal mortality rate was 673 per 100,000. In 2006 about half of all mothers received some kind of antenatal service, and 15% of deliveries were attended by a health worker. Ethiopia has escaped the ravages of HIV/AIDS when compared with other countries in Africa: it had an adult prevalence of 2.1% in 2006.

The WHO (2008) reports that in 2003 there were 1,936 physicians in Ethiopia, representing a population-physician ratio of approximately 38,000, or 0.03 physicians per thousand individuals. This is the fifth highest population to physician ratio among African countries, and compares pitifully with the ratio of 10,000 recommended by the WHO. If anything near this ratio is to be attained, there will clearly need to be a sustained long-term increase in the net supply of physicians to the Ethiopian market. The shortage of nurses is less acute, but similar expansions will be necessary.[1] The recruitment and retention of health workers in both the public and private sectors of the local market depends on the financial and nonfinancial rewards that they expect to reap relative to alternatives (such as non-health sector work or migration). On the other hand, the allocation of a given supply of health workers across geographic regions, as well as to tasks and specialties, often depends on the relative rewards in the public and private sectors. Attracting health workers to remote areas is a particular challenge if the WHO-recommended ratios are to be met in a meaningful way.

Rural and remote areas of Ethiopia are particularly underserved by health workers. We do not have nationally representative data on health worker location by rural and urban areas, but Ministry of Health data indicate that in 2004 about 20% of the approximately 1,000 doctors classified as operating in the "public sector" worked in Addis Ababa, home to about 5% of the population (Ministry of Health 2005). It is likely, of course, that physicians in other regions are also located in urban centers, so the share of public sector doctors in rural areas would be far less than 80%. To add further to this rural-urban disparity, Ministry of Health data suggest that a further 1,500 doctors work for NGOs, other governmental organizations (e.g., the military), the "central" government, and in the private sector. We do not have specific data on their location, but we believe that few of them serve the rural population. By some estimates, half of the physicians in Ethiopia serve the residents of the capital, Addis Ababa.

During the 1980s and most of the 1990s, health workers trained in Ethiopia were typically assigned to their first jobs by the central government. This assignment was by means of a lottery system, and the prevailing belief among officials we interviewed is that the control exercised by the state was such that most health workers accepted their assignments. Workers were required to serve a fixed number of years before being "released" and permitted to apply for other positions. During the past five years Ethiopia has embarked on a radical decentralization program across all areas of the public sector, with much of the responsibility for service delivery being devolved to lower levels of government. In each of the 10 regions, plus Addis Ababa, a regional health bureau has responsibility for the hiring and deployment of public sector health workers.

As competition between regions for health workers has grown, anecdotal evidence suggests that the lottery system has become increasingly ineffective. It is believed that many new graduates do not register for the lottery, and those who do participate are prone to disregard their assignments if they so wish, knowing that they can apply directly to the regional health bureau for jobs. The regions compete on salaries, time to release (which allows work in the burgeoning private sector, at least in Addis Ababa), and other attributes. Some regions, for example Oromia, have recently introduced explicit financial incentives to attract individuals to remote areas *within* the region. Similarly, regions that are themselves remote (in terms of being far from Addis Ababa) have attempted to attract health workers by providing certain training options and financial incentives.

In this paper we estimate health worker preferences over different job attributes in an attempt to identify the factors that are important to health workers in influencing their labor supply decisions. One approach to this problem is to study actual choices made by health workers. However, this method may suffer from a range of selection and endogeneity problems, leading to biased parameter estimates. In addition, there is often limited variation in key job attributes (pay and non-pay), making it challenging to estimate the effects of these parameters on labor market choices and to predict the effects of changes in job attributes that lie outside the existing range over which these attributes vary in practice. Of course, the obvious downside to this approach is that we might have more confidence in choices people actually make than in the choices they might say they would make.

Stated preference techniques have been widely used in health and environmental economics applications to study preferences for nonmarketed commodities. Discrete choice experiments (DCEs) have examined the valuation of different attributes of health care service provision, dimensions of health benefit beyond health outcomes, and quality of care attributes (for reviews see Ryan and Gerrard 2003a and 2003b). Studies of health worker valuations of job attributes have also adopted DCE methods, both in the UK (Scott 2001, Ubach et al. 2003, Wordsworth et al. 2004) and in a variety of low- and middle-income settings (Chomitz et al. 1998; Mangham and Hanson 2007; Penn-Kekana et al. 2005). Chomitz et al. provide a useful review of the benefits and shortcomings of the approach. A study of recent medical and nursing school graduates currently underway in Ethiopia elicits direct measures of the cost of taking a rural job, but does not employ the DCE technique.

Data and DCE Methodology

In this section we report our sampling strategy and the details of the discrete choice experiment we conducted.

Sampling

Our sampling strategy aimed at obtaining representative samples of doctors and nurses from three of Ethiopia's eleven regions—the capital city of Addis Ababa, Tigray, and the SNNPR. Addis is a city of about 3 million people and is located in the central highlands. Tigray has a population of about 4 million people and lies in the extreme north of the country, bordering Eritrea, and the SNNPR, with a population of 14 million borders Kenya to the south. Our sample is representative within these geographic areas.[2] The design over-sampled doctors in the SNNPR and Tigray due to the small number of doctors outside Addis Ababa: all doctors in these rural regions were sampled, while only about one third of doctors in Addis were. Our final sample included 219 doctors and 645 nurses working in health centers and hospitals.

A random sample of one third of doctors was achieved in Addis Ababa by (a) randomly sampling facilities of the various types with sampling weights corresponding to the estimated proportion of doctors working across the different facilities; and (b) interviewing all doctors at the sampled facilities. In the SNNPR and Tigray, all doctors were included in the sample. This was achieved by sampling all public hospitals in the SNNPR and Tigray (there are generally no doctors in non-hospital health facilities in these regions and there were no private hospitals).

A randomly selected sample of approximately one sixth of all nurses was achieved in Addis Ababa by having the enumerators randomly select half of all nurses at the sampled facilities. In the SNNPR and Tigray we (a) randomly selected one sixth of all nurses working in government hospitals; (b) randomly selected one sixth of the sub-regional districts or woredas which have a hospital, visited all health centers in these woredas, and interviewed all nurses in these health centers; and (c) randomly selected one sixth of the woredas without hospitals, visited all health centers in these woredas, and interviewed all nurses in these health centers. Although for logistical and budget reasons (to minimize transport costs) the sample was selected using a cluster approach (with the facility as the cluster), as there is no strong reason to expect health worker preferences within a facility to be correlated we have not adjusted for clustering in the analysis. A summary of our sample is provided in Table 3.1.

Among doctors, the interview response rate varied widely across regions. In Tigray it was very high (88%), while in the SNNPR and Addis Ababa it was lower—58% and 66% respectively. In Addis, the response rates differed in public and private facilities. At public facilities, all doctors present agreed to be interviewed, although 40% of sampled doctors were absent on the day of the interview (28% for unexplained reasons and 12% for planned leave). However at private facilities, no unexplained absences were recorded, although 18% of doctors were absent on planned leave. In contrast to public facilities, the share of

Table 3.1. Facilities and Health Workers Surveyed in Addis Ababa

	Addis Ababa	SNNPR	Tigray	Total
Facilities	40	39	18	97
Hospitals	6	12	11	29
Health centers and clinics	34	27	7	68
Health workers	362	206	293	861
Doctors	91	72	56	219
Nurses	271	221	150	642

sampled doctors who were present but refused to be interviewed was 27%. In Tigray, non-response arose because one sampled facility no longer existed, and one was inaccessible for security reasons, but at visited facilities absenteeism and refusal rates were very low. In the SNNPR, 42% of doctors listed as being employed were absent at the time of the facility visit, although nine out of ten of them were reported as being absent for training purposes.

For nurses, we do not have data on refusals to be interviewed, but we have calculated response rates as the ratio of the numbers of nurses interviewed to our initial target sample.[3] These calculated rates varied by region: in Tigray, nurses at both hospitals and clinics appear to have been over-sampled, leading to an interview rate of 143% (i.e., 43% more nurses were interviewed than initially targeted), whereas in the SNNPR about 70% of the target number were interviewed. Most of the under-sampling seems to have occurred at health centers, which may have been under-staffed compared with our pre-survey estimates. In Addis there was a small degree of over-sampling—the sampling protocol appears to have been followed in hosptials (where 50% of nurses in sampled facilities were to be interviewed), with slight over-sampling in health centers.

Finally, a short facility-level survey was conducted at each hospital or health center that was visited. This survey gathered information on the facility conditions, availability of equipment and medical supplies, etc. The interview was conducted with the director of the facility or another senior administrative officer before the individual questionnaires were administered.

The Discrete Choice Experiment

Each health worker interviewed was presented with a questionnaire with two modules: the first of which solicited factual data on the worker's circumstances, incomes, household characteristics, etc., and the second of which contained a series of hypothetical choices that the respondent was asked to make. The second module provides the underlying data for our discrete choice analysis. We characterized a job in the public sector by discrete values of each of six attributes. These attributes were chosen based on their perceived relevance to health worker decisions in Ethiopia, following discussions with officials from the Federal Ministry of Health and the heads of regional health bureaus in Addis Ababa, Mekele (the capital of Tigray) and Awasa (the capital of the SNNPR). The choice of attributes was also informed by focus group discussions undertaken as part of a similar study in another low-income country in sub-Saharan Africa, Malawi (Mangham and Hanson 2007). The attributes chosen are shown in Table 3.2.

The attribute *values* or *levels* were chosen both to be realistic and to provide a wide enough range of variation to enable predictions about relatively large policy changes to be made. The values of the location attribute differed for doctors and nurses. In practice, very few doctors work outside towns, so for them we allowed the location attribute to be either

"Addis Ababa" or "Regional Capital." For nurses however, this attribute took on the values "City" and "Rural."[4] At the time of the study, public sector health workers were paid on the basis of a pay scale based on experience, qualifications, etc. We used the (unweighted) average monthly salary from these scales to determine a "base" salary for doctors and nurses separately, and let the pay attribute take on values each to 1, 1.5, and 2 times this value. The third (housing), fourth (equipment and drugs), and fifth (time commitment[5]) attributes in Table 3.2 took on the same values for doctors and nurses. For doctors, the final attribute was permission to work in the private sector (taking the values yes and no). Because opportunities for providing nursing services outside regular hours are limited, the opportunity to work in the private sector is of limited use for nurses. However, experience from other countries has suggested that active and supportive supervision is an important job attribute for these health workers. This is the sixth attribute we included for nurses.

Our questionnaire presented individuals with a series of pairs of jobs and asked them to choose the one they preferred from each pair. There are in principle 144 ($= 2 \times 3 \times 3 \times 2 \times 2 \times 2$) distinct jobs charactized by the 6 attributes and hence 20,592 ($= 144 \times 143$) distinct pairs. Using SPSS (Scalable Stream Processing Systems) software, we generated a main effects fractional factorial design with 16 job scenarios. These jobs are shown in Table 3.3. This design satisfies the criteria of orthogonality, minimum overlap and level balance (Huber and Zwerina 1996). To simplify the cognitive task for respondents we elected to use a questionnaire with one job with "middling" attributes as a constant comparator and paired the remaining scenarios to it, giving 15 choices altogether for each respondent. This number of choices is consistent with practice in the health economics literature (Ryan and Gerard 2003a, 2003b).

To examine whether the placement or ordering of scenarios affected responses we administered the questionnaire in four formats. In two of these, the "constant" job was first (on the left-hand-side) in each of the 15 choices, and in the other two it was the second (on the right-hand-side). Similarly, in two formats, the series of 15 pairs were presented in the reverse order. We found no evidence that the questionnaire type had any systematic effect on respondents' answers.

Table 3.2. Job Attributes and Levels

Doctors

Attribute		Possible levels
X^1	Location	Addis Ababa vs. Regional Capital
X^2	Net Monthly Pay (*Base* = 2,500)	1 × Base; 1.5 × Base; 2 × Base
X^3	Housing	None, Basic, Superior
X^4	Equipment and Drugs	Inadequate vs. Improved
X^5	Time Commitment	2 years vs. 1 year
X^6	Private Sector	Yes vs. No

Nurses

Attribute		Possible levels
X^1	Location	City vs. Rural
X^2	Net Monthly Pay (*Base* = 1,250)	*Base*; 1.5 × *Base*; 2 × *Base*
X^3	Housing	None, Basic, Superior
X^4	Equipment and Drugs	Inadequate vs. Improved
X^5	Time Commitment	2 years vs. 1 year
X^6	Supervision	High vs. Low

Table 3.3. The Constant Job, Job 1, and the 15 Comparator Jobs

	Location	Pay	Housing	Equipment and drugs	Time Commitment	Private sector/ Supervision
Job 1	Addis	1.5	Basic	Inadequate	1	Yes/High
Job 2	Addis	1.5	Superior	Inadequate	2	Yes/High
Job 3	Rural	1	Superior	Improved	2	Yes/High
Job 4	Rural	1	Basic	Improved	1	Yes/High
Job 5	Addis	1	None	Improved	1	Yes/High
Job 6	Rural	1.5	None	Improved	2	No/Low
Job 7	Rural	1.5	None	Improved	1	No/Low
Job 8	Addis	1	None	Inadequate	2	No/Low
Job 9	Rural	2	None	Inadequate	2	Yes/High
Job 10	Addis	2	Superior	Improved	1	No/Low
Job 11	Rural	1	Superior	Inadequate	1	No/Low
Job 12	Addis	1	None	Improved	2	Yes/High
Job 13	Rural	1	Basic	Inadequate	2	No/Low
Job 14	Addis	2	Basic	Improved	2	No/Low
Job 15	Rural	2	Basic	Inadequate	1	No/Low
Job 16	Addis	1	Basic	Inadquate	1	Yes/High

Rationality of responses was investigated by including one scenario that was clearly superior to the other, assuming that individuals prefer Addis Ababa (doctors) or urban (nurses) location, higher pay, better housing, more equipment and drugs, shorter time commitment, ability to work in the private sector (doctors), and more supervision (nurses). We found that over 95% of respondents chose the clearly superior job. As it is very possible that some doctors or nurses would have a preference against Addis or urban areas, we chose to retain the full sample of respondents in our analysis.

Specification and Estimation

We label individuals by an index $q = 1, \ldots, Q$. Each potential job is characterized by a set of $a = 6$ *attributes*, and we label the jobs $i = 1, \ldots, 16$. A pair of possible jobs is called (i, j). To motivate our analysis of the data, let $y_{(i,j)q}$ be defined by

$$y_{(i,j)q} = \begin{cases} 1 & \text{if } q \text{ chooses } i \text{ over } j \\ 0 & \text{otherwise} \end{cases}.$$

Let X be an a-dimensional column vector of attribute levels with k th element X^k, and let X_i be the vector of attribute levels that characterize option i. Similarly, let Z_q be a c-dimensional column vector of personal *characteristics* for individual q, with l th element Z_q^l. We hypothesize that individual q derives some utility from option i given by

$$U_{iq} = \alpha + \beta^T X_i + \gamma^T Z_q + \delta \otimes X_i Z_q^T + u_{iq}$$

$$= \alpha + \beta^T X_i + \gamma^T Z_q + \delta \otimes X_i Z_q^T + (e_i + v_q + \varepsilon_{iq}) \qquad (4)$$

where e_i is a job-specific shock, v_q an individual specific shock, and ε_{iq} are uncorrelated shocks, independent of the X s, the Z s, and e_i and v_q. We allow interactions between all pairs of X s and Z s. δ is an (a×c) -dimensional matrix of coefficients with (k, l) th element δ^{kl}, and we define the operation $\otimes$ by $\delta \otimes X_i Z_q^T \equiv \sum_{k=1}^{a} \sum_{l=1}^{c} \delta^{kl} X_i^k Z_q^l$. If we suppose $e_i = 0$, then the difference in utility earned by individual q between options i and j, $\tilde{y}_{(i,j)q}$, is

$$\tilde{y}_{(i,j)q} = U_{iq} - U_{jq}$$
$$= \beta^T (X_i - X_j) + \delta \otimes (X_i - X_j) Z_q^T + \mu_{(i,j)q}. \tag{5}$$

where $\mu_{(i,j)q} = \varepsilon_{iq} - \varepsilon_{jq}$. Notice there is no constant in this expression. We assume then that individual q chooses option i over j (when given this binary choice) if and only if $\tilde{y}_{(i,j)q} > 0$. This occurs with probability

$$P_{(i,j)q} = \text{prob}(\tilde{y}_{(i,j)q} > 0)$$
$$= \text{prob}(\beta^T (X_i - X_j) + \delta \otimes (X_i - X_j) Z_q^T + \mu_{(i,j)q} > 0)$$
$$= \text{prob}(\mu_{(i,j)q} < \beta^T (X_i - X_j) + \delta \otimes (X_i - X_j) Z_q^T)$$
$$= F(\beta^T (X_i - X_j) + \delta \otimes (X_i - X_j) Z_q^T) \tag{6}$$

as long as F(t) prob $(\varepsilon_{iq} - \varepsilon_{jq} < t)$ is such that $f(\,) \equiv F'(t)$ is symmetric about zero. The parameters β and δ are estimated using a random effects probit estimator to capture the within-individual correlation among choices. Where functions of estimated parameters are interpreted, 95% confidence intervals are estimated using the bootstrap method, which has been shown to produce accurate and robust estimates of willingness-to-pay measures (Hole 2007).[6]

Interpretation of Estimated Coefficients

With this specification, individual q's **marginal utility** of the kth job attribute (which, due to our linearity assumption, is independent of the attribute levels associated with alternative i, X_i) is

$$\frac{\partial U_{iq}}{\partial X^k} = \beta^k + \sum_l \delta^{kl} Z_q^l.$$

More meaningfully, the **marginal rate of subsitution** between the k th and h th attributes (which, again, with this specification is independent of the attribute levels associated with alternative i) is

$$MRS_{iq}^{kh} = -\frac{\partial U_{iq}}{\partial X^h} / \frac{\partial U_{iq}}{\partial X^k} \tag{7}$$
$$= -\left(\frac{\beta^h + \sum_l \delta^{hl} Z_q^l}{\beta^k + \sum_l \delta^{kl} Z_q^l} \right)$$

If X^k is pay (i.e., $k = 2$), then the absolute value of MRS_{iq}^{kh} is the marginal value of attribute h to individual q, or individual q's *marginal willingess to pay* for attribute h.

In the special case where Z_q is a binary scalar variable (e.g., sex) taking on the values 0 (male) and 1 (female), the marginal rate of substitution between the k th and h th attributes is

$$MRS_{iq}^{kh} = -\frac{\beta^h}{\beta^k}$$

if $Z_q = 0$ (i.e., for men) and

$$MRS_{iq}^{kh} = -\left(\frac{\beta^h + \delta^h}{\beta^k + \delta^k}\right)$$

if $Z_q = 1$ (i.e., for women).

Attribute Interactions

Under the specification in (4), the marginal rate of substitution between different attributes is independent of the attribute levels (see 7)—that is, indifference curves are straight lines, and the attributes are perfect substitutes. The marginal rate of substitution can be allowed to vary with the mix of attributes by introducing non-linear terms in (4). The simplest way to do this is to include a complete set of interaction terms between the different components of X^i. (We assume that of the interaction terms between attribute levels and individual characteristics, only the linear ones are potentially significant—i.e., there are no terms of the form $X_i^k X_i^h Z_q^l$.) This yields a utility level for person q in job i of

$$U_{iq} = \alpha + \beta^T X_i + \phi \otimes X_i X_i^T + \gamma^T Z_q + \delta \otimes X_i Z_q^T + u_{iq}$$

where ϕ is an $(a \times a)$ upper triangular matrix of coefficients, with (k,h) th element ϕ^{kh}.[7] The difference in utility levels obtained by individual q between jobs i and j is

$$\tilde{y}_{(i,j)q} = U_{iq} - U_{jq}$$
$$= \beta^T(X_i - X_j) + \phi \otimes \left(X_i X_i^T - X_j X_j^T\right) + \delta \otimes (X_i - X_j)Z_q^T + \mu_{(i,j)q}. \tag{8}$$

Following (6), the probability that individual q will choose job i over j is

$$P_{(i,j)q} = \text{prob}(\tilde{y}_{(i,j)q} > 0)$$
$$= F(\beta^T(X_i - X_j) + \phi \otimes \left(X_i X_i^T - X_j X_j^T\right) + \delta \otimes (X_i - X_j)Z_q^T), \tag{9}$$

and the parameters are estimated using maximum likelihood methods for a given assumption about F.

The **marginal rate of subsitution** between the k th and h th attributes is now

$$MRS_{iq}^{kh} = -\frac{\partial U_{iq}}{\partial X^h} \Big/ \frac{\partial U_{iq}}{\partial X^k} \tag{10}$$

$$= -\left(\frac{\beta^h + \left[\sum_{m=1}^h \phi^{mh} X_i^m + \sum_{m=h}^a \phi^{hm} X_i^m\right] + \sum_l \delta^{hl} Z_q^l}{\beta^k + \left[\sum_{m=1}^k \phi^{mk} X_i^m + \sum_{m=k}^a \phi^{km} X_i^m\right] + \sum_l \delta^{kl} Z_q^l}\right)$$

As an example, consider the effect that job location might have on the relative valuation of private practice and money for doctors. The attribue $X^1 = 0$ can take on two values, $X^1 = 1$ if the job is in Addis and $X^1 = 0$ if it is in another city. Similarly, the attribute X^6 can take on two values, $X^6 = 1$ if private sector work is permitted and $X^6 = 0$ if it is not. If we find that the coefficient ϕ^{16} is positive, and that all other $\phi^{kh} = 0$, then the marginal rate of substitution between private sector work and money for a job in Addis is

$$MRS^{26}_{Addis,q} = -\left(\frac{\beta^6 + \phi^{16} + \sum_l \delta^{hl} Z^l_q}{\beta^2 + \sum_l \delta^{kl} Z^l_q}\right),$$

and the MRS between private sector work and pay for a job outside Addis is

$$MRS^{26}_{Non-Addis,q} = -\left(\frac{\beta^6 + \sum_l \delta^{hl} Z^l_q}{\beta^2 + \sum_l \delta^{kl} Z^l_q}\right).$$

Wage Equivalents

We will find it useful to measure the supply response to changes in non-wage attributes in terms of equivalent changes in wage rates. If a change in, say, rural housing is estimated to have a certain impact on rural labor supply, we calculate the change in the rural wage that would have the same quantitative effect on the willingness of health workers to take rural jobs. This sub-section outlines the methodology we employ.

Suppose that a standard or typical job in Addis Ababa is described by a certain bundle of characteristics, X_A, and that the typical rural job is described by a vector X_R. A policy intervention that is aimed at attracting workers to rural areas might improve one or more of the attributes typically found in a rural job, such as improved housing, etc. The vector of attributes defining the average rural job under this policy is denoted X_p. A particular example of a policy intervention involves a change in just the wage earned in rural areas, keeping other attributes at the levels typically found in rural jobs. We think of this policy intervention as an equivalent wage policy. Denote such a vector of attributes by X_E —each component of X_E is the same as the corresponding component of X_R, except for the wage.

These bundles are represented by the following vectors, with the values of the numerical components derived from the survey:

$$X_A = \begin{pmatrix} 1 \\ w_A \\ 0 \\ 1 \\ 2 \\ 1 \end{pmatrix}; X_R = \begin{pmatrix} 0 \\ w_R \\ X^H_R \\ X^E_R \\ X^T_R \\ X^P_R \end{pmatrix} = \begin{pmatrix} 0 \\ w_R \\ h \\ 0 \\ 2 \\ s \end{pmatrix}; X_P = \begin{pmatrix} 0 \\ w_P \\ X^H_P \\ X^E_P \\ X^T_P \\ X^P_P \end{pmatrix}; X_E = \begin{pmatrix} 0 \\ w_E \\ X^H_R \\ X^E_R \\ X^T_R \\ X^P_R \end{pmatrix} = \begin{pmatrix} 0 \\ w_E \\ h \\ 0 \\ 2 \\ s \end{pmatrix}.$$

Note that both h and s will typically vary between doctors and nurses: for doctors, $s = 0$ as there is effectively no private practice in rural areas, but for nurses s represents the prevailing level of supervision that nurses enjoy in rural jobs, which might be non-zero. Similarly, about 40% of doctors in our sample outside Addis report receiving a housing allowance, but less than 10% of nurses in these regions do so (see Table 3.5 below).

The attribute differences between the rural job under the policy intervention and the Addis job are

$$dX_{PA} = X_P - X_A = \begin{pmatrix} -1 \\ w_P - w_A \\ X^H_P \\ X^E_P - 1 \\ X^T_P - 2 \\ X^P_P - 1 \end{pmatrix}$$

while the differences between the rural job with the equivalent wage policy (X_E) and the Addis job are

$$dX_{EA} = X_E - X_A = \begin{pmatrix} 0 \\ w_E - w_A \\ X_R^H \\ X_R^E - 1 \\ X_R^T - 2 \\ X_R^P - 1 \end{pmatrix} = \begin{pmatrix} -1 \\ w_E - w_A \\ h \\ -1 \\ 0 \\ s - 1 \end{pmatrix}$$

In the base attribute-only model, the shares of respondents taking job P over job A, and job E over job A, are respectively

$$P_{PA} = F(\beta^T(dX_{PA})) \text{ and } P_{EA} = F(\beta^T(dX_{EA})).$$

If these are set equal, then $\beta^T(dX_{PA}) = \beta^T(dX_{EA})$, or

$$-\beta^L + \beta^W(w_P - w_A) \quad +\beta^H X_P^H + \beta^E(X_P^E - 1) + \beta^T(X_P^T - 2) + \beta^P(X_P^P - 1)$$

$$= -\beta^L \quad +\beta^W(w_E - w_A) + h\beta^H - \beta^E + \beta^P(s - 1)$$

or

$$\beta^W(w_P - w_A) + \beta^H(X_P^H - h) + \beta^E X_P^E + \beta^T(X_P^T - 2) + \beta^P(X_P^P - s) = \beta^W(w_E - w_A).$$

Alternatively,

$$\Delta w = w_E - w_P$$

$$= \frac{1}{\beta^W} \begin{pmatrix} \beta^H \\ \beta^E \\ \beta^T \\ \beta^P \end{pmatrix} \cdot \begin{pmatrix} X_P^H - h \\ X_P^E \\ X_P^T - 2 \\ X_P^P - s \end{pmatrix}.$$

This is the extent to which a simple wage bonus would need to exceed the wage in the rural bundle to have the same impact on labor supply. Note that in general, the wage equivalent of a policy change that improves a single non-wage attribute will not be the same as the marginal value of, or marginal willingness to pay for, that attribute. This is because the MRS (marginal rate of substitution) between two attributes is calculated holding all other attributes constant, whereas the wage equivalent compares two jobs with different attribute levels.

In a model with characteristic interactions, the same attribute vectors are used, but to find the wage equivalent for a given type of person we now equate the differences in mean latent utilities for that person type. The shares of respondents with characteristics Z taking job P over job A, and job E over job A, are now respectively

$$P_{PA} = F(\beta^T(dX_{PA}) + \delta \otimes dX_{PA}Z^T) \text{ and } P_{EA} = F(\beta^T(dX_{EA}) + \delta \otimes dX_{EA}Z^T)$$

These are equal if

$$\beta^T(dX_{PA}) + \delta \otimes dX_{PA}Z^T = \beta^T(dX_{EA}) + \delta \otimes dX_{EA}Z$$

or

$$\beta^T(dX_{PA} - dX_{EA}) + \delta \otimes \left[dX_{PA} - dX_{EA} \right]Z^T = 0.$$

In the case where Z has just one component, sex, (0 = *male*, 1 = *female*), this reduces to

$$\Delta w_{male} = w_E^{male} - w_R = \frac{1}{\beta^W} \begin{pmatrix} \beta^H \\ \beta^E \\ \beta^T \\ \beta^P \end{pmatrix} \cdot \begin{pmatrix} X_P^H - h \\ X_P^E \\ X_P^T - 2 \\ X_P^P - s \end{pmatrix}$$

for men, and

$$\Delta w_{female} = w_E^{female} - w_R = \frac{1}{(\beta^W + \delta^W)} \begin{pmatrix} \beta^H + \delta^H \\ \beta^E + \delta^E \\ \beta^T + \delta^T \\ \beta^P + \delta^P \end{pmatrix} \cdot \begin{pmatrix} X_P^H - h \\ X_P^E \\ X_P^T - 2 \\ X_P^P - s \end{pmatrix}$$

where δ^W is the coefficient on the wage-sex interaction, δ^H is the housing-sex interaction, δ^E is equipment, δ^T is time commitment, and β^P is private/supervision.

In general, the wage equivalent for individuals with a given characteristic vector is

$$\Delta w(Z) = w_E(Z) - w_R = \frac{1}{\left(\beta^W + \sum_l \delta^{Wl} Z^l\right)} \begin{pmatrix} \beta^H + \sum_l \delta^{Hl} Z^l \\ \beta^E + \sum_l \delta^{El} Z^l \\ \beta^T + \sum_l \delta^{Tl} Z^l \\ \beta^P + \sum_l \delta^{Pl} Z^l \end{pmatrix} \cdot \begin{pmatrix} X_P^H - h \\ X_P^E \\ X_P^T - 2 \\ X_P^P - s \end{pmatrix}$$

where δ^{Xl} is the coefficient on the interaction term between attribute X and characteristic l. If we want to know the wage equivalents for men and women separately, just substitute Z^{sex} = 0 or 1, and use the mean values of the other characteristics in the Z -vector.

Results

Summary Statistics

A summary of facility-level information is provided in Table 3.4. This table includes information provided by a facility administrator in response to a the facility survey, as well as information provided by individual health workers in response to questions about the quality of the facility. Both data sources indicate that workers and patients operate in facilities of generally poor quality, and that on some dimensions at least rural facilities face particular challenges.[8] Private facilities in Addis Ababa tended to perform better on both structural measures of quality and health worker reports of working conditions than public facilities there and in rural areas. Within the public sector, differences between Addis and rural areas are not large, and indeed sometimes favor the rural areas. As well as physical infrastructure, the work environment is conditioned by underlying work practices. One indicator of this is the level of supportive supervision that health workers reported, which, at less than 50%, is rather low.

Descriptive statistics regarding health workers, and indicators of their labor market status, are reported in Table 3.5. In economic terms, doctors in Addis do better than those in the regions. As reported in panel II of Table 35, asset ownership is higher in Addis, with one half and one quarter the doctors working in private and public facilities respectively reporting ownership of a car, compared with less than 2% and 5%, respectively, in the SNNPR and Tigray. House ownership is higher among private sector physicians in Addis (35%), but the rates among other doctors are similar (10–16%). These patterns of asset ownership naturally match the patterns of earned incomes.

Table 3.4. Facility-Level Information, Based on Interviews with an Administrator ("Facility Survey") and Individual Health Workers

Facility survey	All regions	Addis Ababa		SNNPR	Tigray
		Public	Private*		
Number of facilities	77	8	31	21**	17
Reliable elec./phone (%)	92	100	100	97.3	97.6
Functioning laboratory (%)	100	100	100	100.0	100.0
Sufficient water supply (%)	74.2	20.2	96.3	87.2	85.7
Sufficient medicine (%)	78.6	92.5	71.5	88.1	50.0
Sufficient equipment (%)	86.3	87.3	82.6	100.0	69.1

Individual survey (%)	Doc	Nurse	Doc	Nurse	Doc	Nurse	Doc	Nurse	Doc	Nurse
Availability of supplies										
Soap	75.0	69.0	68.7	69.1	100	100	63.8	59.7	53.5	67.1
Water	75.0	75.2	82.5	79.9	98.0	100	59.0	61.8	44.2	77.2
Plastic gloves	88.7	85.7	84.3	84.8	100	100	92.2	84.3	68.6	82.8
Facial mask	58.7	43.0	57.8	51.8	88.9	92.5	49.1	32.1	16.2	23.5
Sterile syringes	93.7	91.8	91.1	92.1	100	100	94.7	92.1	84.4	87.2
Medicines	73.9	70.9	61.3	76.1	97.8	91.3	79.3	73.0	42.2	50.8
Workload										
Often not time to do tasks	55.1	48.2	67.3	58.2	22.0	20.3	82.1	61.2	61.6	31.5
Usually time to do tasks	43.0	51.1	32.7	40.4	72.0	79.8	18.0	38.8	38.4	67.1
Idle time common	2.0	0.6	0.0	1.0	6.0	0.0	0.0	0.0	0.0	1.3
Condition of facility										
Good	43.4	40.9	30.3	24.2	58.0	79.8	39.3	37.0	40.7	46.3
Fair	42.1	45.6	48.5	53.2	38.0	18.6	38.5	51.6	45.4	41.6
Bad	14.5	13.5	21.2	22.6	4.0	1.6	22.2	11.4	14.0	12.1
Supervision										
Supervisor reprimands	31.1	40.3	34.7	39.5	36.0	49.0	34.2	38.8	12.8	38.9
Supervisor supportive	45.3	46.1	32.0	38.3	62.0	68.8	50.4	45.2	26.7	45.0

* Includes for-profit and nonprofit NGO and missionary facilities

** Includes three private facilities.

Doctors working in the public sector in Addis earn salaries about 50% higher than the average doctor in the regions, whereas salaries of private sector doctors are three times as much. Part of this differential likely reflects the return to experience (Addis doctors are older) and specialization (they are more likely to be specialized). However, we find that the rates of specialization in the public and private sectors in Addis are virtually identical, suggesting that training is not the sole driver of observed income differentials. Nurses in Addis earn significantly smaller premiums over regional salaries—about 14% if they work in the public sector and 36% in the private sector.

The gap between private sector salaries in Addis and those of other doctors is partly offset by additional sources of income: public sector doctors in Addis earn additional

Table 3.5. Demographic Characteristics and Incomes of Sampled Health Workers

	Doctors					Nurses				
		Addis					Addis			
	All	Public	Private	SNNPR	Tigray	All	Public	Private	SNNPR	Tigray
Demographics										
Female (%)	18.2	30.0	16.0	2.6	26.7	64.3	73.8	84.4	53.0	61.8
Married (%)	56.6	61.3	74.0	33.3	45.2	63.3	65.3	65.5	50.2	79.3
Age (years)	36.1	39.2	41.2	29.3	31.5	33.4	34.5	35.3	31.0	34.7
	(0.88)	(1.64)	(1.78)	(1.16)	(1.61)	(0.49)	(0.73)	(0.86)	(1.25)	(0.71)
School-aged children in hhld	0.69	0.78	0.82	0.62	0.31	0.94	0.81	0.64	0.93	1.33
Professional										
Primary job priv. (%)	34.9	0.0	100.0	9.4	0.0	14.0	0.0	100.0	5.4	0.0
Ever worked in private sector (%)	46.3	26.6	100.0	14.5	19.8	20.4	24.6	100.0	1.4	8.0
Located in Addis now (%)	60.3					40.0				
Located in regaional capital now (%)	61.9					44.2				
Income										
Salary (US$)	284.5	244.6	480.5	156.4	176.6	100.9	106.8	128.3	87.7	100.8
	(17.4)	(10.5)	(39.0)	(14.8)	(13.9)	(2.0)	(2.1)	(9.6)	(2.7)	(1.96)
Other compensation with job (%)	52.7	29.3	46.0	85.5	53.5	47.0	15.5	35.9	73.3	48.7
Housing (%)	18.9	0.0	0.0	52.1	34.8	5.9	0.0	0.0	11.7	6.7
Total health worker income (US$)	320.9	297.0	496.8	181.4	233.1	102.6	109.3	130.1	87.7	103.7
	(24.8)	(24.8)	(40.1)	(29.7)	(38.2)	(2.1)	(1.7)	(9.5)	(2.70)	(3.7)
Total household income (US$)	443.8	509.2	696.9	196.3	264.3	201.2	298.8	263.9	139.4	157.5
	(28.1)	(49.1)	(55.7)	(30.0)	(46.8)	(12.8)	(22.1)	(25.6)	(10.9)	(10.0)

Figures in parentheses are standard deviations

income equal to 21% of their salaries, while the figures in the SNNPR and Tigray are 17% and 33% respectively, and between one third and one half of doctors in the regions outside Addis report receiving housing allowances (although we do not have data on the monetary value of these allowances). Indeed, significant shares of doctors working outside the Addis private sector report holding more than one job—from 23% in the Addis public sector, to 12% in Tigray. On the other hand, private sector doctors in Addis supplement their (much higher) salaries by only 3%. Although 20% report holding more than one job, we expect that these multiple jobs are in some sense considered together to make up the worker's primary occupation, which accounts for the small amount of supplemental income. Finally, physician household incomes are higher in Addis than elsewhere.

Direct Effects Model

We first estimated a model containing only the direct effects of the job attributes, running this separately on the data for doctors and nurses. The results, shown in Table 3.6, confirm that all job attributes significantly influence job choice in the expected directions. Coefficients and their standard errors are reported for doctors and nurses in the first two pairs of columns. The final pair of columns report the marginal values of each non-wage attribute for doctors and nurses respectively, as a percentage of average base public sector wages (2,500 Birr, or $275, per month for doctors and 1,250 Birr, or $140, per month for nurses). These values are equal to the marginal rates of substitution between the corresponding attribute and pay, as calculated in (7) (with each).

These results suggest that on average, the extra value of a job in Addis relative to one in a regional city for doctors amounts to about one quarter (27%) of the base public sector physician salary, the value of improved housing is about one third (32%), the value of equipment is about one quarter (26%), and the value of reduced time commitment is about one fifth (18%). The most highly prized attribute for doctors is, however, the ability to work in the private sector, which has a value of about half (48%) the base salary.

For nurses the most valuable job attribute is location. Indeed, location appears to be valued more by nurses than by doctors, especially when the value is measured as a share

Table 3.6. The Direct Effects Model, for Doctors and Nurses

	Doctors		Nurses		Marginal attribute value	
Variable	Coef	S.E.	Coef	SE	as % of base salary	
					Doctors	Nurses
Pay × 1000	0.620	0.029	0.992	0.033		
Location	0.415	0.053	0.895	0.031	26.8	72.2
Housing	0.501	0.036	0.582	0.020	32.3	46.9
Equipment	0.409	0.056	0.619	0.033	26.4	49.9
Time commitment	−0.282	0.053	−0.144	0.030	−18.2	−11.6
Private/Super	0.743	0.059	0.404	0.033	47.9	32.6
% correctly predicted	79%		81%			
Log likelihood	−1383.52		−4038.84			
LRT	$p < 0.001$		$p < 0.001$			
n	216		640		216	640

of the base salary. This partly reflects the fact that "location" means something different in the questions nurses were presented with than it does for doctors—switching a job from a rural area, which in principle can be very remote, to a regional capital increases its value by 72% of the base public sector nurse's salary. (The other factor is, of course, the fact that the base nurse salary is only half the base doctor salary.) The least valued attribute for nurses appears to be time commitment, as it is for doctors—having to pay back an extra year after receiving training is equivalent to a pay cut of about 12% of base salary. Improved supervision is valued, but not as highly as the other non-time attributes.

Full Model with Characteristic and Attribute Interactions

We extend the direct effects-only model by incorporating interactions with characteristics that we expect might be correlated with marginal attribute valuations and by including attribute-attribute interactions to assess non-linearities and synergies between attributes. We are particularly interested in exploring which attribute changes are likely to induce individuals to move to a rural posting and which types of people are more likely to respond to a particular policy intervention. The demographic characteristics of greatest interest are marital status, number of children, and sex. We are also interested in the effects on attribute valuation of characteristics of the respondent's *current* job, including its location, housing benefits, and, for nurses, the level of supervision provided.

We adopt a data-driven approach to model construction, in which we first sequentially add interactions of a particular characteristic with pay and non-pay attributes; we then estimate a full model including all the interactions that are individually significant (at the level); finally we remove from this full model all the interactions that are no longer statistically significant (at the $p=0.05$ level). Note, however, that because the and other key model outputs are functions of multiple parameters, some otherwise insignificant interactions are retained in the model in order to calculate standard errors around these functions. Table 3.7 present the results for doctors and nurses.

Our estimates in the full model allow us to examine the heterogeneity of attribute valuations across health workers with different demographic characteristics. Table 3.8 reports selected marginal valuations for doctors, expressed as a percentage of the average base salary of all doctors (2,500 Birr per month). Note that the table includes only marginal valuations of those attributes with statistically significant characteristic interactions.

We find that married doctors value a job in Addis more than three times as highly as single doctors (24% versus 8% of base salary). The most natural explanation for this effect is a combination of joint-career issues and children (although see below on the latter). Also, we see younger doctors place a higher value on reduced pay-back periods following training—at first this seems surprising, as the young have "time on their hands," and we might expect them to be willing and able to pay back more time after training. The result likely arises from the fact that age is confounded with experience and training, so that older doctors, relatively many of whom are already specialized, do not place a high value on the training offered. Alternatively, younger doctors might feel more able to take advantage of their training, say by entering the private sector or seeking future promotions. The future stream of benefits associated with training, even accounting for the length of career over which those benefits will accrue, may be greater for younger, more adaptable, doctors, than for older generations.

The impact of children seems perhaps surprisingly small, particularly the impact of the first child. Doctors with one child value an Addis job (presumably with better schools, etc.) just one percentage point of base salary more than doctors without children, and there is a similarly small difference in the value of housing by number of children. Having a child

Table 3.7. Full Model with Interactions for Doctors and Nurses

Doctors	Coef	S.E.	Nurses	Coef	S.E.
Direct effects			**Direct effects**		
Pay × 1000	0.792	0.116	Pay × 1000	0.816	0.090
Location	−0.367	0.157	Location	0.082	0.103
Housing	0.594	0.051	Housing	0.246	0.048
Equipment	0.535	0.093	Equipment	0.890	0.066
Time commitment	−1.047	0.203	Time commitment	−0.120	0.045
Private/Supervion	0.660	0.088	Private	0.207	0.063
Characteristic interactions			**Characteristic interactions**		
Income × 1000 * location	0.023	0.016	Income × 1000 * location	0.053	0.019
Married * location	0.358	0.124	Married * location	0.011	0.071
Sex * location	0.064	0.146	Sex * location	0.236	0.065
Child * location	−0.025	0.067	Child * location	0.050	0.029
Addisnow * location	0.434	0.119	Citynow * location	0.343	0.074
Sex * pay × 1000	−0.189	0.076	Sex * pay × 1000	−0.179	0.069
Child * pay × 1000	−0.104	0.035	Child * pay × 1000	−0.023	0.031
Married * pay × 1000	0.083	0.069	Married * pay × 1000	0.187	0.076
Age * pay × 1000	−0.006	0.036	Citynow * pay × 1000	0.268	0.071
Sex * housing	−0.009	0.095	Housenow * pay × 1000	−0.398	0.130
Child * housing	−0.059	0.038	Married * housing	0.088	0.042
Sex * equipment	0.129	0.150	Citynow * housing	0.305	0.043
Child * equipment	0.018	0.061	Housenow * housing	−0.145	0.080
Sex * time	0.150	0.143	Married * equipment	−0.091	0.067
Age * time	0.022	0.006	Married * time	0.036	0.062
Child * time	0.006	0.064	Married * supervision	0.069	0.070
Child * private	−0.001	0.065	Private * location	0.173	0.096
Sex * private	−0.148	0.157	**Attribute interactions**		
			Housing * location	0.356	0.065
Attribute interaction			Equipment * location	−0.241	0.075
Private * location	0.484	0.172	Supervision * location	0.291	0.078

increases the value of reduced time commitment following training, but from a relatively small base (13%). These results on the effects of children should, however, be interpreted with caution as the median number of children in our sample of doctors was zero, so extrapolations to larger numbers of children are likely to be imprecise. Nonetheless, taken together with the effect of marriage, they suggest that joint career concerns (and perhaps the *prospect* of children) are more important barriers to rural labor supply than parenthood. Finally, in terms of differences by sex, women are observed to value work in the capital more than men (24% versus 15% of base salary), while men value reduced time commitment about twice as much as women.

Table 3.8. Heterogeneity in Attribute Valuations: Doctors

Characteristic		Marginal attribute value (percent of average base salary)		
		Location	Housing	Time commitment
Age *	24			−25.1
	34.6			−13.3
	40			−7.3
Marital status	Single	7.8		
	Married	24.4		
Number of children	0	16.4	30.3	−13.3
	1	17.4	31.4	−15.0
	2	18.8	33.0	−17.4
Sex	Male	15.3	29.2	−14.0
	Female	24.0	37.5	−7.6

* Ages are the 10th percentile, mean, and 90th percentile.

In contrast, as reported in Table 3.9, married nurses value urban work, and housing, *less* than single nurses. We do not know why marriage should affect nurses' valuations differently to those of doctors. One difference is, of course, that "location" means something different in our estimation of the preferences of nurses and doctors.[9] Married nurses value reduced time commitmnet half as much as singles, suggesting mobility might be more valuable to the latter. The impact of children seems somewhat larger for nurses than doctors (in terms of the percentage of base salary), but again, having children does not seem to be an especially impenetrable barrier to rural work.

Table 3.9. Heterogeneity in Attribute Valuations: Nurses

Characteristic		Marginal attribute value (percent of average base salary)		
		Location	Housing	Time commitment
Marital status	Single	72.8	56.2	−12.2
	Married	59.7	52.6	−6.9
Number of children	0	58.3		
	1	64.2		
	2	70.5		
Income	25th percentile	62.8		
	Mean	63.9		
	95th percentile	69.7		
Lives in a city now	No	58.7	30.3	
	Yes	68.7	45.1	
Works in private sector now	No	61.7		
	Yes	71.9		
Receives housing allowance now	No	53.2		
	Yes	71.3		

Policy Experiments

Our basic policy concern is over what the government can do to induce health workers to take jobs in underserved locations. The specification in (4) allows us to infer the estimated probability of accepting one job (i) over another (j). We use this information in the following section, the impact of attribute changes on rural labor supply, to calculate the probability that a worker will accept a rural job over an urban job and how this probability varies both with other job attributes and across different people. In the section on wage equivalents we convert the effects of job attributes on labor supply to equivalent wage changes by asking what wage change would have the same effect on the probability of accepting a rural job as a given attribute change. Finally, in the section on rural wage bonuses and attributive incentives we illustrate graphically the impact of job attribute improvements on the effect of rural wage bonuses in increasing rural labor supply. Note that in our simulations we do not report the impact of allowing doctors to engage in private sector work outside of Addis Ababa. This is due to the fact that although respondents reported a high valuation of working in the private sector, there are few opportunities to do so outside Addis at this time (although the situation is likely to be changing rapidly), so application of the corresponding coefficients to rural jobs would be misleading.

Impact of Attribute Changes on Rural Labor Supply

First we estimate the impacts of changes in job attributes on the probability that an individual will accept a job in a rural area over a job in Addis Ababa (for doctors) or in a zonal capital (for nurses). For doctors we define job j to be in Addis Ababa, with the prevailing attributes of an average job there set at levels approximating those reported by health workers in the first part of the survey instrument (and similarly for nurses in zonal capitals). Holding public sector wages constant (i.e., without introducing wage bonuses), we calculate the change in the estimated probability of an individual accepting a rural job when one non-wage attribute is improved. The results of this exercise are reported in Table 3.10. Our point estimates indicate, for example, that about 7.5% of doctors would be willing to take a rural job over a job in Addis under prevailing conditions, if they had the choice. Providing incentives in the form of superior housing increases the chance of accepting a rural job to more than one-in-four, whereas provision of basic housing and training incentives (measured by a reduction in time commitment to one year) have relatively small effects, each increasing the likelihood from 7.5% to about 11%. The effect of improving the availability of equipment is in the middle of the range, increasing the probability of choosing a rural job to 17%.

For nurses, the non-wage attribute with the single biggest impact on the share of workers willing to take a rural job is the provision of adequate equipment. At baseline

Table 3.10. Impact of Non-Wage Attribute Improvement on Probability of Accepting a Rural Job, for Doctors and Nurses

	Doctors			Nurses		
	p	95% CI	Increase	*p*	95% CI	Increase
Baseline	0.074	(0.024,0.081)	—	0.046	(0.024,0.050)	—
Basic housing	0.109	(0.040,0.117)	47%	0.097	(0.062,0.107)	112%
Superior housing	0.269	(0.122,0.279)	262%	0.192	(0.142,0.233)	319%
Equipment	0.167	(0.104,0.208)	125%	0.198	(0.147,0.219)	332%
Time commitment	0.114	(0.040,0.136)	53%	0.056	(0.032,0.068)	22%
Equip & housing	0.226	(0.146,0.274)	204%	0.323	(0.273,0.356)	605%
Supervision	—	—	—	0.075	(0.040,0.086)	64%

levels, only 4.4% of nurses would choose a rural job over a city job, but this jumps to 20% if they can be guaranteed adequate levels of equipment. Supplying basic housing, reducing time commitment, and providing better supervision have substantially smaller effects on the probability of choosing a rural job, increasing it to levels in the range of 5% to 8%.

Wage Equivalents

Without information on the costs of making attribute improvements it is difficult to use this information for decision-making purposes. One step in that direction is to calculate the rural wage increases that would yield equivalent labor supply responses for each attribute improvement considered. For example, we ask how much rural wages would need to be increased, holding current non-wage attributes fixed, to induce the same increase in the number of doctors willing to take a rural job that we found for each attribute improvement in Table 3.10. Using the full model estimates reported in Table 3.7, we calculate these wage equivalents (as percentages of the base salary) for men and women separately, as discussed in the sub-section "wage equivalents," under the section on specification and estimation. The 95% confidence intervals around the estimated wage equivalents (again measured in percent of base salary) are bootstrapped in light of the fact that the quantities of interest are non-linear functions of the underlying parameter estimates. The results are presented in Table 3.11 for doctors and nurses separately. A striking result is that although the point

Table 3.11. Wage Equivalents for Doctors and Nurses by Gender

		Doctors						
	Male				**Female**			
	W.E. (% base)		p (rural)		W.E. (% base)		p (rural)	
	Est.	95% CI	Est.	95% CI	Est.	95% CI	Est.	95% CI
Baseline			0.080	(0.025,0.088)			0.050	(0.004,0.097)
Basic house	11.7	(8.9,11.9)	0.116	(0.042,0.128)	12.3	(9.6,19.6)	0.077	(0.016,0.173)
Superior house	45.2	(34.4,46.0)	0.280	(0.130,0.303)	47.3	(36.9,75.7)	0.213	(0.050,0.353)
Equipment	24.6	(21.7,37.1)	0.169	(0.103,0.204)	35.7	(27.2,69.6)	0.157	(0.073,0.264)
Time commitment	14.1	(11.2,13.7)*	0.125	(0.045,0.148)	7.1	(−11.0,28.0)	0.065	(0.011,0.154)
Equip & house	36.2	(31.3,47.9)	0.228	(0.141,0.271)	48.0	(39.8,86.2)	0.216	(0.099,0.352)

		Nurses						
	Male				**Female**			
	W.E. (% base)		p (rural)		W.E. (% base)		p (rural)	
	Est.	95% CI	Est.	95% CI	Est.	95% CI	Est.	95% CI
Baseline			0.063	(0.047,0.078)			0.038	(0.018,0.044)
Basic house	44.1	(38.2,51.6)	0.126	(0.100,0.152)	53.7	(44.0,62.0)	0.084	(0.050,0.095)
Superior house	92.6	(80.2,108.3)	0.237	(0.189,0.285)	112.7	(93.5,131.5)	0.171	(0.121,0.205)
Equipment	57.4	(47.9,67.0)	0.244	(0.207,0.281)	69.9	(58.8,80.5)	0.176	(0.126,0.199)
Time commitment	8.0	(1.7,14.3)	0.076	(0.056,0.095)	9.8	(2.1,17.1)	0.048	(0.025,0.060)
Equip & house	101.5	(86.5,118.5)	0.380	(0.337,0.423)	123.6	(107.1,142.3)	0.294	(0.242,0.331)
Supervision	31.3	(24.4,39.9)	0.099	(0.074,0.124)	38.2	(30.9,47.0)	0.064	(0.032,0.076)

Notes: Due to bootstrap bias, the point estimate may lie outside the estimated CI. This occurred once in our simulations (*).

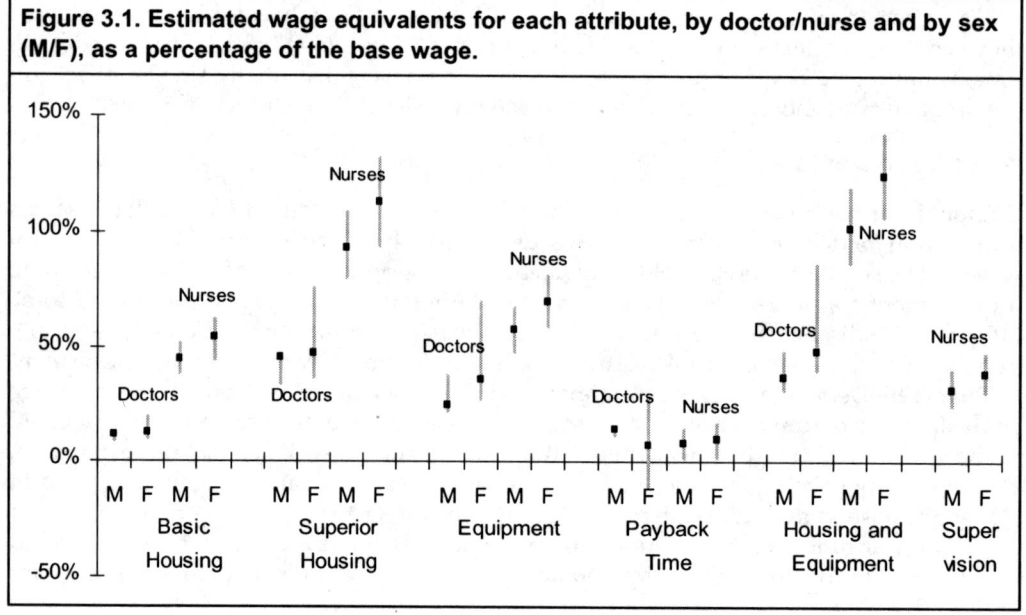

Figure 3.1. Estimated wage equivalents for each attribute, by doctor/nurse and by sex (M/F), as a percentage of the base wage.

estimates of wage equivalents for all attributes are higher for women (except when it comes to the value doctors place on time commitment), the difference is never statistically significant. This is illustrated in Figure 3.1.

Rural Wage Bonuses and Attribute Incentives

Finally, we investigate the impact of increases in rural pay on predicted health worker labor supply based on our regression results. In particular, we estimate the probability that an individual will accept a rural job as a function of the excess of pay over the base pay rate. This is the most obvious way to induce greater labor supply, but we also calculate the impact of such wage increases when coupled with attribute improvements. The results, for doctors and nurses respectively, are presented graphically in Figures 3.2 and 3.3, respectively. For doctors, doubling pay while keeping other attributes constant increases the probability of accepting a rural job from 7% to 57%. Alternatively, to induce half of doctors to locate in rural areas under current conditions, a rural bonus of approximately 89% (2,225 Birr) is required. Providing basic housing does not affect the impact of wages to a large extent, probably because most doctors already have at least basic housing. On the other hand, providing superior housing means that doubling wages increases the probability of accepting a rural job from 27% to 84%.

Our results suggest that nurses are much less responsive to proportionate wage bonuses than doctors—a doubling of pay increases the probability of accepting a rural job from 4% to only 27%, and inducing half of the nursing workforce to locate in rural areas would require a wage bonus of about 155% of the base salary. This bonus amounts to 1,937 Birr, and is only marginally smaller than that needed to induce a similar proportion of doctors to take jobs in rural areas. The impact of adequate equipment, both on willingness of nurses to take a rural job in itself and on the impact of higher pay on such willingness, is of particular interest, especially because this attribute does not reflect personal consumption as such. Indeed, the impact of equipment is not only greater than that of basic housing, but it exceeds that of *superior* housing also. By itself, adequate equipment increases the likelihood of accepting a rural job from 4% to 21%, and when coupled with a doubling of rural pay this probability increases to 61%.

Figure 3.2. Share of doctors willing to accept a rural job as a function of the rural wage bonus (horizontal axis), with alternative in-kind attribute incentives.

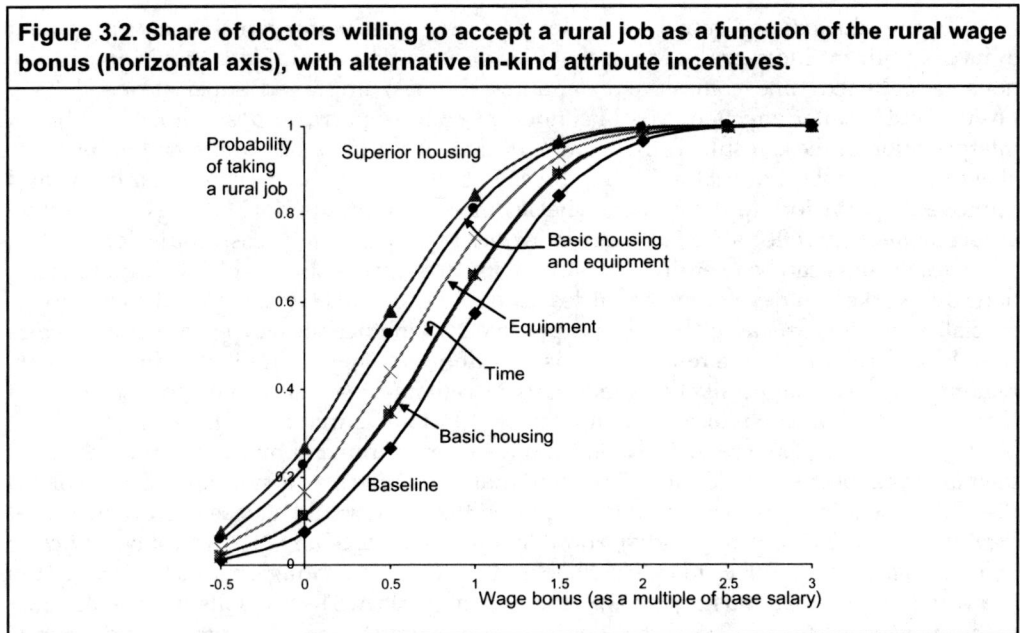

Conclusions

Our analysis provides evidence that the locational labor supply decisions of health workers are responsive to both wage and non-wage factors, and that for some of these attributes the responses can be large. Proportionate wage bonuses for rural service increase labor supply, but these effects seem to be larger for doctors than for nurses. For example, under current working conditions in urban and rural facilities, attracting 50% of doctors to work in regional towns would require a wage bonus of approximately 89% over the base salary. Inducing the same rural labor supply from nurses to rural settings (which are on average more remote than regional towns) would require a bonus of about 155%.

Figure 3.3. Share of nurses willing to accept a rural job as a function of the rural wage bonus (horizontal axis), with alternative in-kind attribute incentives.

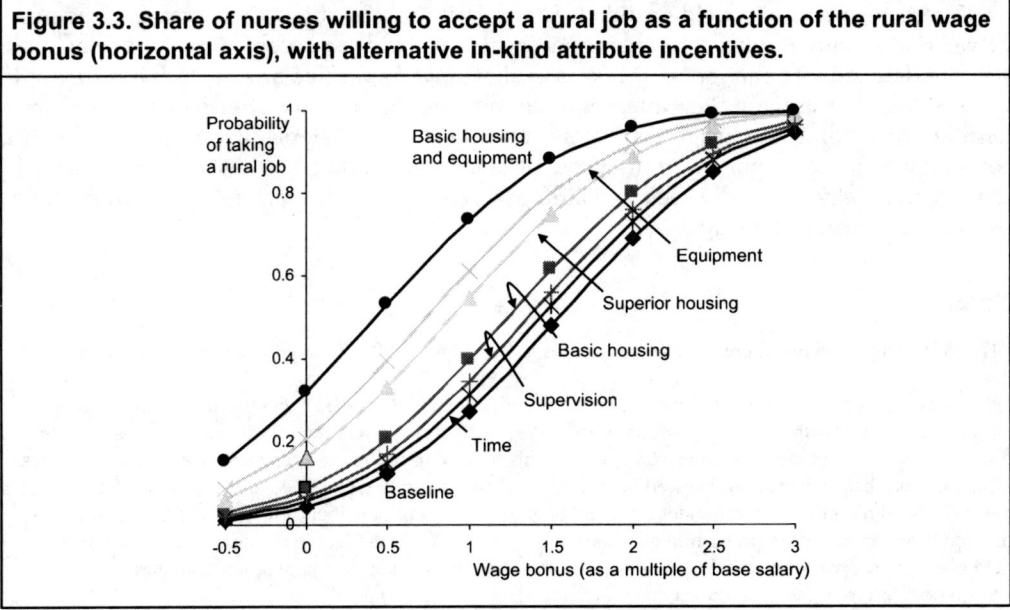

For both doctors and nurses, the joint provision of superior housing *and* equipment induce significant increases in the probability of accepting a rural job. Provision of basic housing, reduced time commitment, and (for nurses) improved supervision all have positive but smaller effects on the likelihood of choosing a rural post. Our broad-brush interpretation of these results is that health workers want to be paid more and to be better able to do their jobs, but that in-kind inducements in the form of accelerated training and improved supervision are valued somewhat less. The fact that superior housing is an effective inducement likely reflects the fact that this would represent a large cash equivalent.

These results can be usefully compared with two similar studies of stated preferences of health workers in developing countries. Chomitz et al. (1998) found that the promise of specialist training was an effective, if expensive and inefficient, way of inducing doctors from Java to relocate to the remote islands of Indonesia. They found that individuals *from* remote areas were more likely to take jobs *in* remote areas, and that modest financial incentives could induce relocation to moderately (but not extremely) remote areas.

Serneels et al (2005) report results from a survey of nursing and medical students in their final year of study in Ethiopia. They find that at the then prevailing starting wage of 700 Birr, fully one third of nursing students reported that they would choose to work in a rural area (defined as 500km from Addis), and that a rural bonus of just 31% would be sufficient to induce *all* student nurses to take such jobs. To get all graduating doctors to move to the rural areas requires a bonus of just 39% of the starting salary. These results stand in contrast to those of this paper: we found that doctors in our sample would need to be paid a bonus of about two and a half times the base salary in order to induce (nearly) all of them to work in a rural area, and the corresponding figure for nurses is about three times the base salary. The difference may stem from the fact that our samples were very different: Serneels et al. interviewed students, whereas we surveyed health workers at various stages of their careers. Finally, Serneels et al. report that the availability of children's educational opportunities was one of the main attractions of work in Addis Ababa. Somewhat surprisingly, we find only weak evidence of this effect in our data: the number of school-aged children a health worker has does not appear to have an economically significant influence on her or his valuation of alternative job attributes (including location). We speculate that this may be due to the widespread practice of sending children to boarding school amongst Ethiopia's upper classes.

These results can provide guidance to policy-makers about the potential trade-offs between alternative policies to encourage health workers to accept rural jobs. However, without detailed information on the costs of altering the specified attributes, it is impossible to rank the alternative policy interventions in terms of any cost-effectiveness measure.[10] On the other hand, our wage-equivalent analysis is a first step toward allowing such a comparison. In addition, the limitations of stated preference studies should be kept in mind, and ideally we would seek to validate our results by comparing them with evidence from revealed preference analyses.

Notes

[1] The WHO estimated that there were 14,270 nurses in Ethiopia in 2003, or about one nurse for every 5,250 people.

[2] Other regions, such as Oromia (which surrounds Addis Ababa) and Amhara (which is immediately north of Oromia) are larger (with 26 and 19 million residents respectively) and less remote, at least in terms of direct distance measures, but we have no reason to expect this to have introduced systematic biases in our estimates.

[3] The total number of nurses interviewed in each region was determined by budgetary constraints. Following this, and based on pre-survey estimates of the number of nurses working at each facility, the data firm was provided with an estimated proportion of nurses to be interviewed at the facilities (but could revise this in the field if the pre-survey estimates did not match the actual size of the regional population of nurses).

[4] A full description of the instructions given to respondents is in the appendix.

[5] Time commitment refers to the number of years that an individual is required to work at an institution per year of further training sponsored by that institution, after the training is completed.

[6] We constructed the bootstrapped confidence intervals manually by calculating 100 estimates of the relevant variable and reporting the simple averages of the 2nd and 3rd percentiles as the lower limit and those of the 97th and 98th percentiles as the upper limit. The alternative method is to assume normality and to calculate the limits of the confidence interval as the estimate plus/minus 1.96 times the estimated standard deviation of the 100 repetitions. However on a number of occasions this method produced negative lower bounds for a probability variable, indicating that the distribution of the bootstrapped estimates was not close to normal.

[7] $\phi^{kh} \geq 0$ for $k \geq h$ $\phi^{kh} = 0$ for $k < h$.

[8] The facility administrators paint a somewhat rosier picture of conditions than do workers. Our interviewers did not independently verify conditions as reported by the administrators: we could speculate that their relatively positive evaluations might have been due to strategic misreporting (due to a sense of pride perhaps), or due to incomplete information (if the administrators did not face the realities of poor working conditions on a daily basis).

[9] Perhaps it is more important for single nurses to be in a city "marriage market" than it is for single doctors.

[10] Note that cost-effectiveness is a useful measure if the objective of increasing labor supply is taken as given. It does not inform the question of whether such changes in labor supply are warranted— we take this as self-evident in this case.

References

Anand, Sudhir, and Barnighausen, Till. 2004. "Human Resources and Health Outcomes: Cross-Country Econometric Study." *Lancet* 364 (9445):1603–9.

Chomitz, Kenneth, Gunawan Setiadi, Azrul Azwar, Nusye Ismail, and Widiyarti. 1998. "What Do Doctors Want? Developing Incentives for Doctors to Serve in Indonesia's Rural and Remote Areas." Policy Research Working Paper 1888, World Bank, Washington DC.

Hole, A. R. 2007. "A Comparison of Approaches to Estimating Confidence Intervals for Willingness to Pay Measures." *Health Economics* 16 (8): 827–40.

Huber J., and K. Zwerina. 1996. The Importance of Utility Balance in Efficient Choice Designs." *Journal of Marketing Research* 33: 307–317.

Joint Learning Initiative. 2004. *Human resources for health: overcoming the crisis.* Boston MA: Joint Learning Initiative.

Mangham, L., and K. Hanson. 2007. "Eliciting the Employment Preferences of Public Sector Nurses: Results from a Discrete Choice Experiment in Malawi." Unpublished mimeo.

Ministry of Health, Government of Ethiopia. 2005. *Health and health-related indicators: 1997.*

Penn-Kekana, L., D. Blaauw, K. S. Tint, D. Monareng, and J. Chege. 2005.: "Nursing Staff Dynamics and Implications for Maternal Health Provision in Public Health Facilities in the Context of HIV/AIDS." Johannesburg: Centre for Health Policy, University of the Witswatersrand.

Ryan, M., and K. Gerard. 2003a. "Using Discrete Choice Experiments in Health Economics: Moving Forward." In *Advances in Health Economics*, eds. A. Scott, A. Maynard, and R. Elliot, t John Wiley and Sons.

Ryan, M., and K. Gerard. 2003b. "Using Discrete Choice Experiments to Value Health Care Programmes: Current Practice and Future Research Reflections." *Applied Health Economics and Health Policy* 2 (1): 55–64.

Scott, A. 2001. "Eliciting GPs Preferences for Pecuniary and Non-pecuniary Job Characteristics." *Journal of Health Economics* 20: 329–347.

Serneels, Pieter, Jose Garcia-Montalvo, Magnus Lindelow, and Abigail Barr. 2005. "For Public Service or for Money: Understanding Geographical Imbalances in the Health Workforce." Policy Research Working Paper 3686, World Bank, Washington DC.

Ubach C., A. Scott, F. French, M. Awramenko, and G. Needham. 2003. "What Do Hospital Consultants Value about Their Job? A Discrete Choice Experiment." *British Medical Journal* 326: 1432–1438.

WHO. 2006. *World Health Report 2006: Working together for health.* Geneva: World Health Organization. http://www.who.int/whr/2006/en/

WHO Global Atlas of the Health Workforce. http://apps.who.int/globalatlas/default.asp

Wilbulpolprasert, S., and P. Pengpaibon. 2003. "Integrated Strategies to Tackle the Inequitable Distribution of Doctors in Thailand: Four Decades of Experience." *Human Resources for Health* 1: 12.

Wordsworth, S., D. Skatun, A. Scott, and F. French. 2004. "Preferences for General Practice Jobs: A Survey of Principals and Sessional GPs," *British Journal of General Practice* 54 (507): 740–746.

Eco-Audit

Environmental Benefits Statement

The World Bank is committed to preserving Endangered Forests and natural resources. We print World Bank Working Papers and Country Studies on postconsumer recycled paper, processed chlorine free. The World Bank has formally agreed to follow the recommended standards for paper usage set by Green Press Initiative—a nonprofit program supporting publishers in using fiber that is not sourced from Endangered Forests. For more information, visit www.greenpressinitiative.org.

In 2008, the printing of these books on recycled paper saved the following:

Trees*	Solid Waste	Water	Net Greenhouse Gases	Total Energy
289	8,011	131,944	27,396	92 mil.
*40 feet in height and 6–8 inches in diameter	Pounds	Gallons	Pounds CO_2 Equivalent	BTUs

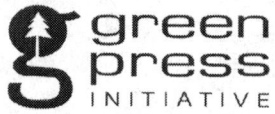
green press INITIATIVE